Training Manual for Total Parenteral Nutrition

AUTHOR:
Richard E. Dean, M.D.
Professor and Chairman, Department of Surgery
Michigan State University, East Lansing, MI
Former Director, Metabolic Nutritional Support Service
Butterworth Hospital, Grand Rapids, MI

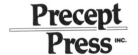

Precept Press INC.

94   5   4   3   2

Library of Congress Catalog Card Number:
90-62754

International Standard Book Number:
0-944496-18-0

Precept Press, Inc.
160 East Illinois Street
Chicago, Illinois 60611

Printed in the United States of America

Total Parenteral Nutrition

Table of Contents

Historical Introduction to Intravenous Nutrition

Physicians have long been concerned about nutrition, acknowledging the importance of nutrients in man for maintaining lean body mass, intact immune systems, wound healing, and prevention of complications. Intravenous hyperalimentation can trace its roots to 1656 when Sir Christopher Wren[1] utilized the first known intravenous administration set. Crude in design, the set was composed of a goose quill attached to a pig's bladder to introduce ale, opium, and wine into dogs' veins. In 1831 Thomas Latta[1] first successfully used the mode of parenteral therapy to treat the intractable diarrhea of his patients with cholera. Sixty years later, Rudolph Matas[1] utilized the same solution as a treatment for surgical shock in man.

By the end of the 1800's, the intravenous use of glucose for nutritional purposes had begun. This concept was not pursued, however, until 1911 when Kausch[1] reported the use of intravenous glucose in a patient following surgery. Fat emulsions as IV nutrients in dogs were used several years later by Murlin and Riche,[1,2] and later applied to man by Yamakawa.[1,3]

The 1930's saw intravenous infusions enter into a new area of patient care. Cuthbertson[1] defined the metabolic needs of patients following severe trauma and initiated the use of protein hydrolysate in the intravenous solutions. Rhoads and his associates[1] significantly accelerated the progress of intravenous nutrition during World War II by administering higher levels of protein and calories to patients post-operatively. The result was nitrogen equilibrium. By 1942, solutions containing three major nutrients—carbohydrates, protein, and fat—were administered intravenously to provide nutrition to adult patients. However, complication of delivery and patient intolerance limited the usefulness of these early products.

The feasibility of central venous infusion was recognized in the early 1950's by a French surgeon, Aubaniac,[3] who introduced subclavian venipuncture as a means of rapidly administering blood to battle casualties in the French Indochina War. Subclavian venipuncture had been practiced for some time in this country, but it was not until Dudrick and his associates applied this technique to TPN that it achieved its present popularity. In 1965, Dudrick, Rhoads, and Vars[1,2] demonstrated that solutions containing essential amounts of amino acids, dextrose, vitamins, and minerals could support the growth and development of weanling puppies being fed entirely by vein for a minimum of ten weeks. After this success, the method was applied to humans. Parenteral diets were successfully formulated for adults and infants as a result of Dudrick's success. An intravenous means of providing calories and proteins was now available for patients whose lean muscle masses had wasted due to illness.

Parenteral nutrition had progressed to the point where the long-term needs of critically ill patients were being addressed. In 1969, Scribner, Broviac, and associates[1,2] realized that an arteriovenous shunt, previously used only for hemodialysis, could also provide easy access for the delivery of total parenteral nutrition at home. This concept of longterm parenteral nutritional support, known as Home Parenteral Nutrition (HPN), has now achieved the function of "an artificial gut."

In the short frame of time since TPN was developed, its utility, wide-ranging application, safety, and life-saving abilities are now widely accepted.

This book was prepared to help physicians find the answers to TPN questions without going through a lot of trouble and pages. If you refer to the expanded table of contents, you should be able to locate answers and references to questions and problems that may come up at the bedside. Tables and References follow chapter nine. As you will note, the book fits easily into a lab coat pocket, and we hope that physicians, especially residents and interns, will want to keep it there.

You will find that the systems and techniques we describe really work. They were developed and refined at Butterworth Hospital, Grand Rapids, MI. Since their introduction at Butterworth in 1977, complications associated with subclavian catheters have fallen from 15% to less than 1%.

1/Patients Who May Benefit from TPN

When considering total parenteral nutrition (TPN), a number of questions must be answered, including which patients need nutritional support and how to select those who would benefit from TPN acknowledging the risk factors and costs involved. In consideration of these issues, certain groups of patients are at high risk of nutritional depletion with its attendant high complication and mortality rates. These patients are frequently grouped in the categories listed below:

1. _Surgical Complications:_ Patients with intestinal fistulas or obstruction following surgery and those with problems originating from intraabdominal complications, including abscess with local or generalized peritonitis, will usually require aggressive nutritional support to achieve a satisfactory outcome.

2. _Pre-op Preparation:_ Patients undergoing major operations will commonly demonstrate evidence of moderate to severe malnutrition as a result of the underlying disease process. Classically, patients with esophageal or upper gastrointestinal obstruction will present for operation with marked weight loss, deficient visceral protein, and other stigmata of protein-calorie malnutrition.

3. _Gastrointestinal Diseases:_ Patients with malabsorption syndromes or acute exacerbations of chronic

inflammatory bowel disease, such as ulcerative colitis and Crohn's disease, may benefit from bowel rest and aggressive parenteral nutrition. Likewise, patients with inflammatory bowel disease who have undergone extensive medical therapy will demonstrate the catabolic effects of steroids in addition to the inadequate absorption and poor assimilation of nutrients due to their disease.

4. _Organ Failure:_ Patients with renal and hepatic failure can improve significantly with appropriate attention to nutritional needs. Pulmonary failure, a problem of increasing proportions, is commonly accompanied by major nutritional deficits requiring judicious nutritional support to help resolve infection and provide the energy necessary for ventilatory weaning.

5. _Anorexia:_ This problem, commonly associated with cancer, chemotherapy, and irradiation, is also identified in patients with neurologic disorders such as multiple sclerosis, degenerative diseases, and cerebral vascular accidents. Anorexia nervosa is yet another problem associated with significant nutritional deficiencies.

6. _Hypermetabolic States:_ Burned, traumatized, or septic patients generally require intensive nutritional support.

2/Identifying the Malnourished Patient

Specific identifying characteristics of malnutrition are needed to focus on those patients who will benefit from aggressive nutritional support. The increased risk of morbidity and mortality in the malnourished patient will more than justify the risk, cost, and time expenditure needed to correct the nutritional deficit. Although numerous nutritional assessment parameters have been described and avidly supported, only a few are readily available and commonly used.[4]

1. *Rapid weight loss:* A 10% weight loss within 6-8 weeks indicates a significant loss of lean body mass, giving rise to increased morbidity and mortality. Similarly, patients admitted with weights 10% below their ideal weight may have limited reserves which are readily depleted by infection, trauma, or surgery. *A rule of thumb in determining ideal weights* which has proven to be quite effective, is as follows: The ideal weight for a woman five feet in height is 100 pounds, and 5 pounds are added for each additional inch. The ideal weight for men 5 feet tall is 106

pounds, and 6 pounds are added for each additional inch. These estimated ideal weights are considered accurate within 10%.[4]

2. *Serum albumin* levels below 3.0 grams per deciliter indicate depleted protein reserves which are associated with a higher morbidity and mortality.[5]

3. *Five to ten days of NPO status* seriously jeopardizes metabolic reserves and increases the risk of complications. Patients with minimal dietary intake for several days or those ingesting nothing by mouth (NPO) should alert the clinician to potential nutritional deficiencies which may call for an aggressive TPN program.[4]

4. *Serum transferrin* can be used effectively to predict the protein-calorie status of a patient.[6,7] The 8 day half-life of this iron-transport protein makes it particularly vulnerable to inadequate nutrition or catabolic states. Because of these characteristics, serum transferrin is equally useful in predicting an improved nutritional status and should show a definite rise in patients receiving adequate nutrition along with proper control of the disease process. Albumin, because of its long half-life (20 days) and its variability due to hydration and capillary permeability, has limited usefulness in monitoring the nutritional repletion of deficient patients.

5. *Total lymphocyte counts* (WBC x the percent lymphocytes) may be useful as an indicator of nutritional deficiencies. However, the variability of the total lymphocyte count due to infection and immune-suppressed states induced by steroids, chemotherapy, radiation therapy, and tumor, reduces its relia-

bility. Thus, as a nutritional assessment parameter, it must be used with caution in those groups of patients. Total lymphocyte counts less than 1500 in patients without infection or immunosuppression are highly suggestive of nutritional problems, and those with counts of 800-1000 are at great risk of increased morbidity and mortality. Although the total lymphocyte count has been used effectively in assessing patients on admission, our experience indicates that is has questionable value when monitoring in-hospital patients because of frequent infection and the liberal use of steroids, antibiotics, and other drugs, many of which have cytotoxic effects on the lymphocytes or their precursors. The total lymphocyte count has, therefore, been of little use as a tool to monitor in-house patients for nutritional deficiencies or to follow their nutritional status once started on a support program.

3/Standard Techniques

Consultation

Once the patient at high risk for malnutrition is identified, a thorough assessment of the patient is necessary to determine the extent of the problem and to develop a plan of action. In Butterworth Hospital, this task is completed at consultation. A standardized consultation form (Figure 1) has been in use for several years and has proven to be an effective tool. The consult form consists of several sections, the first of which includes all of the patient identification data, including name, age, date of admission, and hospital number. The inclusion of these data aids greatly in retrieving patient charts needed for clinical study at later dates.

The second section of the consultation form includes a brief list of the patient's problems and would include such data as the problems leading to admission, date of operative procedures, and list of complicating factors. The dietary history section explores the patient's dietary habits and allows the examiner to make critical assessments regarding the adequacy of the oral intake in the

METABOLIC NUTRITIONAL SUPPORT SERVICE CONSULTATION   Date _____

Patient Name _____ Number _____ Age _____ Sex _____

Hospital _____ Room _____ Adm. Date _____ Marital Status _____ Race _____

Physician _____ Adm. Complaint _____

Current Diagnosis and Problems _____

_____

_____

_____

_____

Nutritional Assessment:
Diet History, including days NPO _____

_____

Current medication:
Steroids _____ Vitamins _____ Alcohol _____

Antibiotics _____ Chemotherapy _____ Minerals _____

Other _____

Weight Loss: Wt. 6 mos. ago _____ 3 mos. ago _____ Adm. wt. _____ Present wt. _____

Laboratory: Admission   Most recent   Admission   Most recent

	Admission	Most recent			Admission	Most recent
Tot. Prot.	____	____	WBC		____	____
Albumin	____	____	RBC		____	____
Na	____	____	Hbg		____	____
K	____	____	% Lymph		____	____
Cl	____	____	Total Lymph		____	____
CO_2	____	____	ProTime		____	____
BUN	____	____	Liver Func.		____	____
Creatinine	____	____	Other		____	____

Nutritional Requirement:

Height _____ Ideal Weight _____ lbs. = _____ kgs Calorie load _____ cals/kg

Recommended Calories _____ Recommended Protein _____

PLAN: _____

_____

_____

_____

_____

_____

_____

_____   _____
                                     Signature   Date

Revised 11/79

Figure 1: Standard Consultation Form.

weeks, days, or months preceding the consultation.

This section is followed by a list of commonly used drugs, i.e. steroids, antibiotics, chemotherapy, and alcohol, many of which have profound catabolic effects or other influences on nutrition which may affect the plan of management. The medical section is followed by a recall of weights at 6 months, 3 months, and on admission, as well as the most recent recorded hospital weight.

A comparison of admission laboratory data to those on the date of consultation is then listed on the consult form. Of particular interest are the total proteins, albumin, electrolytes, BUN, creatinine, and liver function tests. Additional space is provided for other laboratory data which may be especially pertinent to the patient.

Establishing the Nutritional Plan

The section on nutritional requirements, listed at the bottom of the consultation form, is an important element in the nutritional consultation. The previously recorded data will have demonstrated the extent of the nutritional deficiency, and will provide other information essential to the choice of nutritional support method to be recommended.

Caloric Requirements

Determination of nutritional requirements focuses primarily upon caloric need. Indirect calorimetry measurements of energy utilization in numerous groups of patients receiving TPN in our institution have been compared to the standard Harris-Benedict equation, Long's modification of the Harris-Benedict equation, the Wilmore nomogram, and the rule of thumb 35 calories per kilogram per 24 hours.[8,9] Results of these studies indicated that caloric (non-protein) requirements closely approximated the Harris-Benedict equation, or 25 calories per kilogram per 24 hours, irrespective of the stress state (Table I). All calculations were based on ideal body weight using the rule of thumb standard previously described. Without indirect calorimetry methods of determining basal metabolic expenditure (resting energy equivalent), 25 calories per kilogram of ideal body weight should be used as the recommended non-protein caloric load. Using this method, the patient's ideal weight in pounds divided by 2.2 will convert the weight to kilograms. The kilograms are then multiplied by 25 calories to determine the recommended daily non-protein calorie requirement for the patient.

Protein Requirements

Proteins are usually administered at a rate of 1 gram per kilogram per 24 hours. Septic and stressed patients may require protein concentrations in excess of 1.5 grams per kilogram per 24 hours. Patients with hepatic failure may require restrictions of protein due to the metabolic impairments in converting ammonium to urea.[2,10] Patients with liver problems or an elevated bilirubin are frequently started at 20 grams of protein per 24 hours and gradually advanced to higher concentrations as their clinical status dictates. Patients with renal failure may require strict limitations of protein, depending upon the degree of renal failure.[11-14] Special renal failure solutions have been developed and will be described later.

Vitamins, Trace Minerals, Essential Fatty Acids

All patients receiving nutritional support will require adequate vitamin replacement. Additional vitamins are probably indicated as most patients seen in consultation are significantly malnourished. Trace minerals in the form of zinc, copper, manganese, and chromium should be infused with the TPN solutions daily.[15,16] Deficiencies in zinc or copper should be appropriately treated. Lipids are required to prevent essential fatty acid deficiencies. This objective can be achieved by the infusion of 500 ml of 10% lipid emulsion two times per week. Patients with diabetes or who are intolerant to the high glucose levels delivered in TPN may benefit from the use of continuous infusions of lipid to provide up to 50% of the non-nitrogen calorie source.

Using this information, a nutritional plan can be developed for the patient, including the route of administration and the recommended non-nitrogen calories, proteins, vitamins, and trace minerals to be provided. Additional comments may be necessary to highlight any special problems which might be anticipated during treatment with the aggressive nutritional support program proposed.

Placement of the Central Venous Catheter

Although other vascular access techniques are available, the most commonly used method remains the percutaneous subclavian venipuncture. The advantages of this method over the internal jugular or supraclavicular approach depends upon individual preference, ease of catheter care, and patient comfort. Placement of a subclavian catheter to be used for total parenteral nutrition requires careful consideration of the following factors.[17-21]

1. Examine the neck, anterior chest, both shoulder areas, and upper arms. Numerous engorged subcutaneous veins extending from the upper shoulder or supraclavicular area to the neck or anterior chest may provide the only clue to an occult subclavian vein thrombosis. Patients who have been chronically ill, repeatedly hospitalized, or those who have undergone aggressive supportive care with Swan-Ganz catheters or previous central venous lines should be suspected of having a deep vein thrombosis. A recent subclavian puncture site, hematoma, edema, or erythema should alert the clinician to potential problems which may have been encountered with previous subclavian catheterization attempts. Acute subclavian vein thrombosis is identified by the presence of edema in the supraclavicular fossa, extending onto the anterior chest and upper arm with accompanying engorgement of the superficial veins of the upper arm, forearm, and hand.

2. Identification of structural abnormalities of the thoracic inlet and clavicular area may eliminate one or both subclavian veins from consideration for catheter placement. Examples of such problems might include a distorted clavicle as a result of recent fractures or remote injuries, tumor masses in the supraclavicular area, or recent incisions from biopsy sites. In addition, patients having prosthetic devices such as axillary-femoral extra-anatomic arterial bypass, peritoneal venous shunt (Laveen or Denver shunt), and those with transvenous pacemakers carry undue risks of injury to the prosthetic conduit to justify placement of the subclavian catheter on that side.

3. Assessing the state of hydration is an essential clinical skill which is frequently overlooked.[22] Attempting to place a subclavian catheter in a volume-depleted patient is fraught with complications and frequently associated with an unsuccessful attempt. Placing the patient in supine or even Trendelenburg position can provide a quick assessment of the intravascular volume. Examining the mucous membranes, conjunctiva, and axilla for moisture, tenting the skin over the anterior chest and abdomen, and reviewing the intake and output records will further clarify the patient's state of hydration.

4. Review of the medication record for evidence of anticoagulation may provide significant information. Patients on therapeutic heparinization programs or on Coumadin require the utmost in planning and coordination with the primary physicians to allow for subclavian catheterization when anticoagulant effects are at a minimum. Review of laboratory data on trauma or tumor patients will frequently identify abnormal coagulation profiles, i.e. prolonged protime or inadequate platelet count. Correction of these coagulation parameters may be required before attempting subclavian catheterization. Occasionally, these risks must be assumed and the catheter placed in a most expeditious manner. Under these circumstances, the patient, family, and primary physicians should be informed of the increased risks and appropriate component blood therapy made available. Alternative routes of central venous catheterization should also be considered in these situations. Placement of a long-arm catheter

or a cephalic vein cutdown may be attendant with reduced risk to the patient with bleeding problems.

Preparation for Subclavian Catheterization

Knowledge of the subclavian procedure, including familiarity with the venous anatomy, subclavian catheter technique, and the equipment required, is essential to the safe placement of the subclavian catheter. A subclavian catheter insertion kit, carefully prepared to include all necessary equipment and supplies, is the basic ingredient required for a low-risk TPN system (Figure 2). This insertion kit should provide the solution necessary for preparing the skin, sterile gloves to be used during skin preparation, and additional sterile gloves to be used by the clinician and the assistant during catheterization. It should also include syringes, needles, local anesthetic, ointments, and dressings. Sterile towels, catheters, extension tubing, IV solution and the appropriate monofilament suture with a needle driver or hemostat and scissors complete this kit (Figures 3-6). The use of this approach eliminates the risk of contamination while waiting for needed supplies or equipment to arrive from the nearest supply depot.

Successful placement of the catheter depends primarily upon maximizing your potential for hitting the subclavian vein. Improved hydration will increase the intravascular volume and ultimately provide for venous distention, which will expand the target and improve your odds of hitting the vein. When possible, a peripheral IV should be started 12-18 hours prior to the procedure and run at a rate sufficient to accomplish this objective. Usually, this will entail starting an IV in the late afternoon at a

Figure 2: Catheter Insertion Kit supplies.

SUBCLAVIAN CATHETER KIT

Amount	Supply
4 pair	Sterile procedure gloves, size medium
3 pkgs.	Sterile drapes
4	Masks
1 liter	D5W
1 pkg	Solution administration set
1 pkg	Extension tubing
2	6cc syringes
1 each	Needles: 21 gauge and 19 gauge
1 bottle	1% xylocaine
1 bottle	Freon TA
1 bottle	Tincture of benzoin
1	14 gauge Bard intracath
1 pkg	4-0 nylon suture
2 pkgs	10% Betadine solution
1 pkg	Betadine ointment
2 pkgs	10x14 cm Opsite bandages
1 roll	2-inch paper tape
7 pkgs	4x4 gauze
4 pkgs	2x2 gauze
1	Suture removal set

Figure 3: The first part of the subclavian catheter kit includes: 1 liter D5W, 1 solution administration set, 2 pair size medium sterile procedure gloves, 1 bottle Freon TA, 1 pkg. Povidine solution, 3 pkgs. 4x4 gauze sponges.

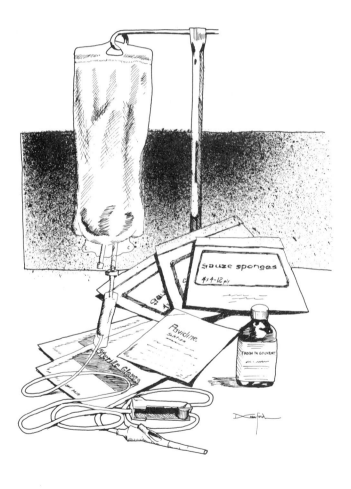

Figure 4: The second part of the subclavian catheter kit includes: 3 pkgs. sterile drapes, 1 bottle 1% xylocaine, 1-6 cc syringe, 1-19 gauge needle, 1-21 gauge needle, 1 pair size medium sterile procedure gloves.

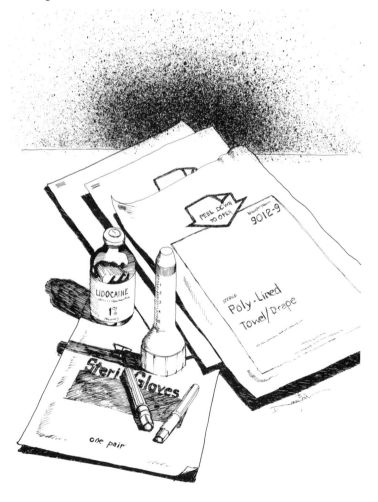

Figure 5: The third part of the subclavian catheter kit includes: 1-14 gauge Bard intracath, 1 pkg. extension tubing, 1-6 cc syringe, 1 pkg. 4-0 nylon suture, 1 suture removal kit, 1 pkg. povidine solution, 1 pkg. 4x4 gauze sponges.

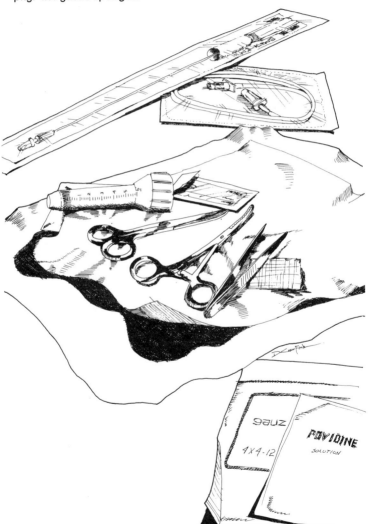

Figure 6: The fourth part of the subclavian catheter kit includes: 1 bottle Tincture of Benzoin, 4 pkgs. 2x2 gauze sponges, 2 pkgs. 4x4 gauze sponges, 2 pkgs. 10x14 cm. Op-Site, 1 pkg. povidine-iodine ointment, 1 roll 2 inch paper tape.

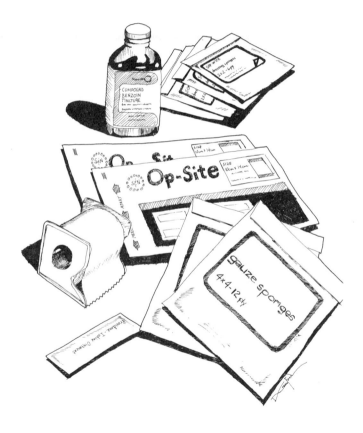

rate of 125-200 ml/hour using Ringer's lactate or D5/half normal saline to adequately hydrate the patient for placement of the catheter at 8:00 a.m. the next morning. Better hydration has contributed greatly to our improved success rate in achieving subclavian vein catheterization from 85% in 1975 to 94% in 1980 when a more aggressive fluid replacement program was instituted.

Intravenous sedation with meperidine (Demerol) and diazepam (Valium) has proved to be an extremely useful adjunct to successful placement of the catheter. Usually, 50 mg of Demerol given IV slowly, supplemented with 2.5-5 mg of Valium given in a similar fashion, allays patient anxiety and reduces patient restlessness which can lead to contamination of the sterile field. This premedication frequently produces patient amnesia of the procedure. Lower doses and occasionally elimination of the IV sedation may be indicated, particularly in the very brittle or acutely ill patient. A reversing agent (Narcan) should be available since apnea, requiring reversal of the narcotic, has occurred in 3 of our past 500 subclavian catheterizations. Following hydration and sedation, the patient should be placed in Trendelenburg position.

Placement of the Subclavian Catheter

Under ideal circumstances, the right subclavian vein is the preferred side because of its more direct route to the superior vena cava, especially when using an 8″ catheter. Withdrawing the catheter to attach the needle guard over the 2-inch needle places the catheter tip at the level of the junction of the superior vena cava with the right atrium (Figure 7). When approached from the left, the 8″ catheter tip frequently lays at the junction of the brach-

Figure 7: Ideal placement of the subclavian catheter occurs on the right side and places the catheter tip at the level of the junction of the superior vena cava with the right atrium.

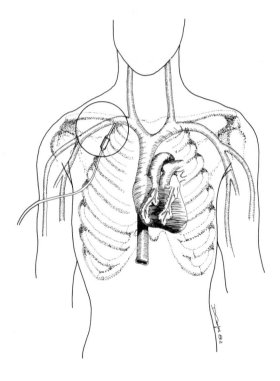

iocephalic vein and the superior vena cava when withdrawn sufficiently to protect the needle. The right subclavian vein offers the further advantage of eliminating
any potential injury to the thoracic duct, located at the
junction of the internal jugular and subclavian veins on
the left. However, should the anatomy of the right clavicular area be distorted or the risk high, due to other
factors previously listed, the left subclavian vein should
be approached without hesitancy.[17-21]

A folded towel or sheet is placed longitudinally beneath the thoracic spine to allow the shoulders to fall
back, providing room to direct the needle between the
clavicle and first rib. This is especially important when
performing the procedure in the patient's bed. This ma-
neuver may not be necessary when performing the catheterization on hard surfaces such as an x-ray table, operat-
ing room table, or procedure table. The patient's head
should be turned in the opposite direction to reduce
airborne contamination of the area. The physician and
assistant should apply face masks and sterile gloves. The
subclavian area selected for inserting the catheter should
be cleansed gently with a non-flammable degreasing
agent such as Freon TA. The prep area should include the
base of the neck, supraclavicular area, and anterior chest
extending across the midline. A Povidine-iodine solution
prep is then applied to the previously degreased area,
using gentle friction. After a second Povidine-iodine
prep to the same area, the physician should change
gloves and apply drapes to isolate the subclavian area,
supraclavicular fossa, and anterior chest.

In an attempt to reduce the complications associated
with subclavian catheterization and develop a teaching

method which could be used with residents, medical students, and other inexperienced clinicians, we have developed the "Walk-Off Technique" for subclavian vein catheterization. This method emphasizes three distinct steps:

1. The apex of the costoclavicular groove is identified (Figure 8).
2. A skin wheal is formed with lidocaine 1 cm below the clavicle and 2 cm lateral to the apex of the costoclavicular groove. A 1.5-inch 22-gauge needle is walked off the clavicle in a line perpendicular to the long axis of the clavicle (Figure 9). The needle is then advanced 1 cm beneath the clavicle in the same perpendicular line.
3. The needle is redirected towards the superior margin of the manubrium sternum (Figure 10). This redirection of the needle is accomplished by movement of the mobile skin and subcutaneous tissue without advancing or withdrawing the needle. The needle is advanced in a plane, parallel to the anterior chest and immediately below the level of the sternum (1 cm), until venous blood is withdrawn. Local infiltration of the tissues with lidocaine is then accomplished, and the needle is withdrawn. A 14-gauge needle is positioned on the syringe so that the needle bevel corresponds with the syringe numbers. The large bore needle is advanced in the same, precise manner as the infiltrating needle, advancing through all three steps previously listed.

If unable to enter the subclavian vein with initial advancement of the needle and gentle aspiration, the needle is withdrawn approximately 1 inch and redirected

Figure 8: The shaded area represents the costoclavicular groove. The needle puncture site is 1 cm. below the clavicle and 2 cm. lateral to the apex of the costoclavicular groove.

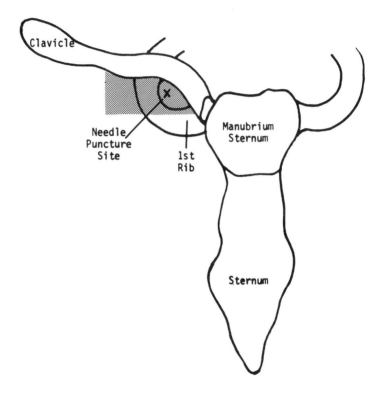

Figure 9: The needle is walked off the clavicle in a line perpendicular to the long axis of the clavicle, then advanced 1 cm. beneath the clavicle in the same perpendicular line.

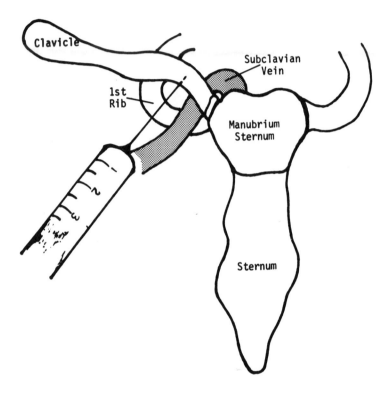

Figure 10: The needle is redirected towards the superior margin of the manubrium sternum, then advanced in a plane, parallel to the anterior chest and immediately below the level of the sternum (1 cm.), until venous blood is withdrawn.

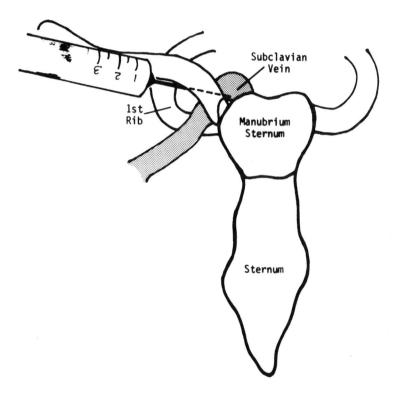

cephalad 1 cm to the level of the suprasternal notch in the same superficial plane. If again unsuccessful, the needle is withdrawn 1 inch and redirected approximately 1 cm cephalad in the same plane. Failure to penetrate the subclavian vein in this superficial plane calls for a redirection of the needle 1 cm deeper into the midplane (Figure 11). This is best accomplished by withdrawing the needle, using the same skin puncture site, but walking off the clavicle lateral to the initial attempt. Moving laterally on the clavicle 1.5-2 cm drops the needle into a deeper plane (midplane) without incurring the risk associated with angling the needle such that penetration of the artery is likely. At this plane, the needle is again advanced to the level of the superior margin of the manubrium sternum and redirected 1 cm cephalad with each unsuccessful attempt. Dropping to a deeper level (deep plane) can usually be accomplished by moving laterally on the clavicle through the same skin perforation. At this deeper level, the risk of entering the artery becomes significant, and the most experienced clinician should be engaged to repeat the walk-off technique, using the three needle advancements in each plane before entering the deeper planes of the thoracic inlet. Particular attention should be paid to maintaining a line of needle advancement which is directed at right angles to the midline or slightly inferior (towards the heart), as advancing the needle in a more cephalad manner will direct the catheter into the internal jugular vein rather than the superior vena cava.

Assuming that the vein has been punctured, the needle is advanced 0.5 cm, and free flow of venous blood is ascertained by withdrawing and injecting the blood. The needle and syringe are then rotated so that the bevel is

Figure 11: Thoracic Inlet (Sagittal Section):
    A: Superficial Plane. 1 cm below sternum
    B: Mid Plane. 2 cm below sternum
    C: Deep Plane. 3 cm below sternum.

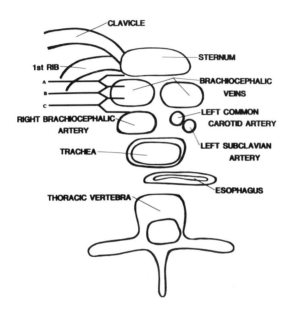

now facing inferiorly (towards the heart) and again, blood must be drawn in and out of the syringe freely.

The gloved assistant attaches a hemostat to stabilize the needle hub, the syringe is loosened, and the catheter advanced into the superior vena cava. Occasionally, difficulty is encountered when attempting to pass the catheter beyond the 14-gauge needle. Although the easy access of blood would indicate that the needle is within the lumen of the vein, advancing the catheter may be difficult, if not impossible. Under these circumstances, the catheter stylus should be withdrawn 1-2 cm and passage of the catheter again attempted. If the catheter has been advanced beyond the needle tip but does not pass readily into the vein, it is advisable to remove the entire catheter and needle as a unit to reduce the hazard of shearing the catheter tip.

Upon placement of the catheter, the needle catheter unit is withdrawn so that the needle is outside of the skin. The catheter is connected to the sterile extension tubing loaded with D5/half-normal saline and the IV infusion opened full bore to verify patency in a large vein. The needle catheter guard is attached, taking care to assure that no blood is trapped within the needle guard. The area is generously swabbed with Povidine-iodine solution. The infusion bag is lowered below the level of the patient to insure a rapid reflux of blood up the IV tubing. The IV bag is then hung on the IV stand, and the rate adjusted to prevent overloading. The catheter is secured in place with a 4-0 monofilament nylon suture. The suture is passed through the skin and subcutaneous tissues superior and medial to the puncture site, and the suture is tied over a hemostat to insure a loose attachment to the skin. The suture is then passed over and around the catheter and tied securely to the catheter at the skin exit site. No further attachments of the catheter or needle guard to the skin are necessary, as extensive suture could enhance bacterial growth and would reduce mobility of the catheter during dressing changes. A small dab of Povidine-iodine ointment is applied at the catheter exit site and an Opsite dressing applied after painting the skin with tincture of benzoin. The Opsite dressing should include the entire catheter and 1-2 inches of the connector tubing. Firm adherence of the Opsite to skin and tubing must be assured at completion of this procedure. A loop of extension tubing should be securely taped to the dressing, and the dressing dated and initialed by the surgeon or assistant.

The catheter insertion procedure is incomplete until the patient's chest has been examined for equal breath sounds and a chest x-ray obtained to confirm proper placement of the catheter without evidence of pneumo-thorax (Figures 12 and 13).

Automatic Aborts of the Subclavian Catheterization Procedure

Subclavian artery penetration with a 14-gauge needle or catheter should signal a halt to all further proceedings, since the risk of developing additional complications increases dramatically due to the presence of the resultant hematoma. Arterial injuries requiring operation because of hemorrhage, entimal flaps, or thrombosis are rare, but the potential merits close observation with repeated hemoglobin/hematocrit monitoring and clinical observation for vascular insufficiency. A second complication

Figure 12: X-Ray confirms proper placement of the subclavian catheter.

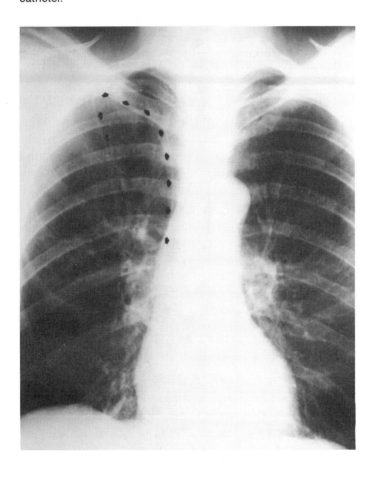

Figure 13: X-Ray shows that pneumothorax has occurred in catheterization attempt. Immediate management of the pneumothorax is the primary concern.

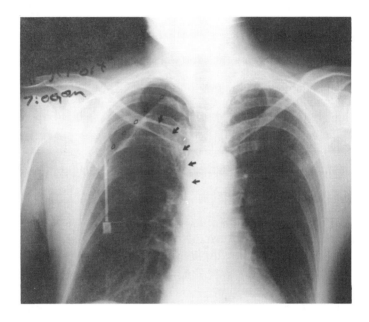

requiring the immediate cessation of all further catheterization attempts occurs with the free aspiration of air signalling a pneumothorax. An immediate chest x-ray and appropriate management of the pneumothorax should be the primary concern.

The Unsuccessful Subclavian Catheter Attempt

In our experience, failure to successfully place the subclavian catheter occurs in approximately 6% of all subclavian catheter attempts. Our initial failure rate in 1977 was 12% (Table II). This rather high failure rate can be attributed to inexperience with the technique and lack of attention to details such as hydration and careful evaluation of the patient for occult venous thrombosis. Failure to accept defeat seems to be the single most significant factor responsible for some of the major complications associated with subclavian catheterization. The random blind probing of the thoracic inlet with a 14-gauge needle can prove to be costly to the patient, demoralizing to the clinician, and devastating to a nutritional support effort. A planned approach using the "Walk Off" technique and a systematic probing of the anterior plane of the thoracic inlet should prove adequate. Further random probings can be associated with disaster.

A specific plan of action should be initiated following an unsuccessful subclavian catheter attempt:

1. Examine the patient for evidence of pneumothorax or neurovascular injury;
2. Obtain a chest x-ray to rule out an unrecognized pneumo- or hemothorax;
3. Re-examine the patient to insure that an occult

venous thrombosis has not been overlooked; and
4. Reassess the patient's state of hydration.

Usually a more vigorous hydration program is indicated and appropriate measures should be initiated to correct the problem. At this point, a decision must be made whether an alternative route for central venous catheterization, i.e. a long-arm silastic catheter, cephalic vein cutdown, or placement of a Hickman catheter under direct vision would be advisable. Obtaining a venogram may prove useful in identifying an aberrant venous drainage system. Although any of the above central venous access options may be satisfactory or even desirable, a more common approach is to make appropriate plans for subclavian catheterization on the opposite side 18-24 hours later. Prior to proceeding with a catheter placement procedure on the opposite side, the patient must be carefully re-examined to insure that a delayed pneumothorax has not developed.

The Misdirected Subclavian Catheter

Approximately 5% of all subclavian catheters will be misdirected into the internal jugular vein or opposite subclavian vein, making them unacceptable for the infusion of TPN (Figures 14 and 15). Although acceptable for the infusion of isotonic solutions or medications, misdirected catheters will initiate a venous thrombosis when hypertonic TPN solutions are infused into these low flow systems. It is mandatory that all intravenous catheters placed with the purpose of infusing TPN be placed in the superior vena cava where high blood flow rates reduce this hazard. In an effort to eliminate the unnecessary risk

Figure 14: Catheter misdirected into the internal jugular vein.

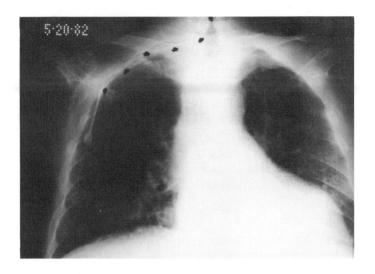

Figure 15: Catheter misdirected into the opposite (Left) subclavian vein.

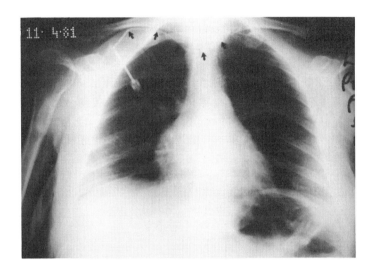

of pneumothorax or vascular injury associated with subclavian catheter placement, we have adopted a technique of manipulating all misdirected catheters under
fluoroscopic visualization (Figure 16). This procedure requires little time, minimal patient risk, and insures that
the catheter is in proper position at completion of the
procedure. Our technique involves the following steps:

1. The patient is placed on the x-ray table, the dressing
   is removed, and the catheter area is reprepped and
   draped as in the subclavian catheter placement
   procedure.
2. Under fluoroscopy, a guidewire is advanced through
   the catheter into the venous system. The catheter is
   then withdrawn approximately 2-3 inches.
3. The guidewire is manipulated so that the tip is directed into the superior vena cava. The catheter is
   then advanced and the guidewire withdrawn.
4. IV infusions are reestablished, and the catheter is
   securely sutured in place and the Opsite dressing is
   applied.

In critically ill patients and in those patients on ventilators and other support systems which make it impossible
to transport them to the x-ray department, the catheter
also can be redirected at the bedside using the guidewire
technique and repeated x-rays. The risk of radiation ex-
posure to patients and members of the team should be
minimized. Body shielding with protective aprons is a
requirement for all personnel involved in this procedure.
Rarely is it necessary to perform a second subclavian
catheterization when this technique is used.

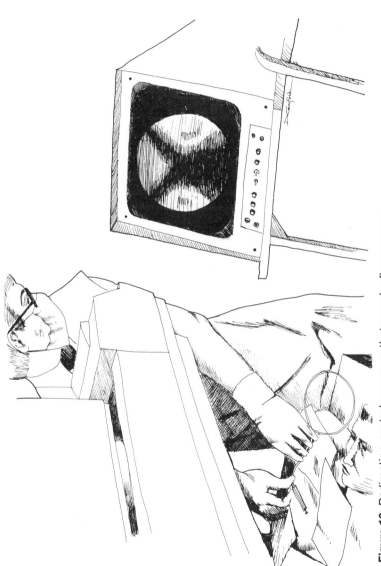

Figure 16: Redirecting central venous catheter under fluoroscopy.

Fever Protocol

Elevated temperatures in patients receiving TPN are not an uncommon occurrence. Usually, the fever can be attributed to an underlying disease process, such as pneumonia, intraabdominal abscess, urinary tract infection, or other causes that may have initially precipitated the need for TPN. The well-entrenched concepts that central venous catheters and TPN are associated with sepsis may be justified in those institutions without a nutritional support program or dedicated personnel. With an active nutritional support service, risk of catheter-related sepsis should not exceed 1%. Thus, patients who develop a fever while receiving TPN may not require immediate removal of the central venous catheter unless the need for TPN is resolved. In those patients in whom TPN must be continued, random removal and replacement of the central venous catheter may be attendant with greater risk of catheter-related complications than sepsis. For these reasons, a fever protocol should be well thought-out and available for implementation.

Patients on TPN who develop a spiking temperature greater than 101 degrees and those with persistently elevated temperatures ranging from 100-101 degrees without an obvious septic source should be carefully evaluated for catheter-related sepsis. Physical examination with particular attention to wounds, hidden abdominal abscesses, and pulmonary infections is the initial step in this evaluation process. Appropriate culture of wounds, drain sites, urine, and other areas which may have been identified as problems during the physical examination should be completed. The TPN dressing should be removed and the catheter site examined under aseptic conditions. Identification of cellulitis or purulence at the catheter exit site calls for immediate removal of the catheter and culturing the exudate. In the event that an obvious catheter-related infection is not present, sterile dressings are applied, and TPN is continued. A spiking temperature occurring immediately after hanging a bottle or bag of TPN solution may herald the existence of a contaminated solution. If this occurs, the bag and IV tubing should be replaced with a D10 solution and new tubing. Samples of the TPN solution should be sent for culture and the bag and tubing returned to the pharmacy for filtering and culture in an effort to concentrate and recover any bacterial contamination.

Most commonly, an inciting factor responsible for the fever will not be identified on initial examination, even though strong suspicion may be directed at a wound, abdomen, or lungs. Twenty-four hours later, the patient should be re-examined, all culture results reviewed to determine the presence or absence of bacterial growth, and the catheter site aseptically examined. If the septic source remains unidentified, blood cultures are drawn through the central venous catheter and a decision must be made regarding removal of the catheter or changing over a guidewire. Unless definite evidence of catheter-related sepsis is identified (purulence or cellulitis at the catheter site), all catheters are changed using a guidewire technique. This decision is based on our early experience with catheters in which positive catheter cultures were rare and a remote septic source was usually identified within 1-2 days. Restarting TPN via a newly-placed subclavian catheter involves considerable risk. One of our early studies (Table II) indicated that 12.2% of all subclavian catheterization attempts were unsuccessful, 6.1% of the catheters were misdirected, and pneumothorax occurred in 6.1%. These complications, which approach 25%, far exceed the 2% catheter sepsis rate. Thus, preservation of the venous access site until the catheter site is proven to be the septic source has been our operational standard. We have followed these guidelines since 1978 and find that, armed with the knowledge that catheters can be changed without complication, subclavian catheters are changed much more liberally. Patients with recurrent fevers may have their catheter changed over a guidewire on multiple occasions during the course of TPN. However, in patients with persistent septic courses without an identifiable source, the catheter should be removed, a peripheral IV started, and a new subclavian catheter inserted 24-48 hours later.

The concern that changing the catheter over a guidewire will reseed the catheter with infection has not been justified in our experience. If rigid catheter care protocol is maintained, hematogenous spread from occult septic sources, i.e. intraabdominal abscess, is probably the most common source of catheter infections. Frequent changing of the subclavian catheter using the guidewire technique may benefit this group of patients and eliminate the risks associated with repeatedly performing subclavian venipuncture.

The Guidewire Technique

A subclavian catheter kit containing the necessary skin preparation solutions, dressings, gloves, masks, catheter, guidewire, and instruments is necessary if the catheter is to be changed in an aseptic manner. The patient is placed flat in bed and the dressing removed. The sterile equipment and supplies are prepared, and an IV and extension tubing are available for use. After carefully cleansing the pericatheter area, gloves are changed, the restraining suture is divided, and the catheter is withdrawn approximately 2 inches (Figure 17). The catheter is divided immediately distal to the needle guard and approximately 8 inches of the guidewire are advanced through the remaining catheter (Figure 18). The catheter is then removed and the tip cultured. The guidewire is liberally swabbed with Povidine-iodine prep solution (Figure 19), and the new catheter passed in over the guidewire (Figure 20). The guidewire is removed, and the catheter is aspirated to insure patency (Figure 21). After reflux of blood has been accomplished, the fluid-loaded connecting tubing is attached to the catheter, the IV is hung and the rate adjusted. The catheter is secured in place with one 4-0 nylon suture and a sterile dressing applied. TPN can be resumed immediately following this procedure. Chest x-rays for catheter position may be obtained if any problems are encountered or doubt exists.

Starting TPN

Confirmation of proper catheter placement by x-ray signals initiation of a TPN plan. Previously prepared consultation forms will have identified the caloric need, protein requirements, and replacement program for vitamins and trace minerals. Writing orders to initiate a plan should include provisions for careful monitoring of the

Figure 17: After removing the restraining suture, the catheter is withdrawn approximately 2 inches and cut immediately distal to the needle guard.

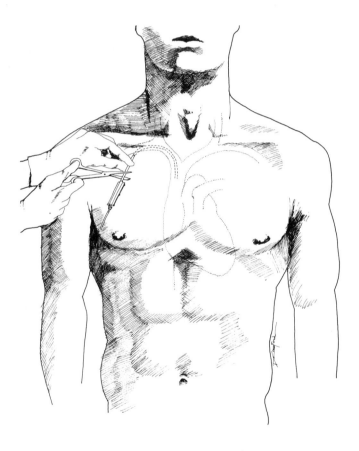

Figure 18: Approximately 8 inches of the guidewire is advanced through the remaining catheter.

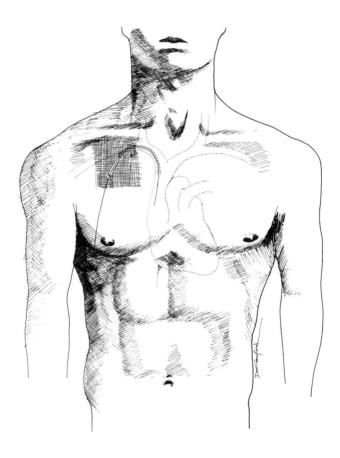

Figure 19: The guidewire is liberally swabbed with the povidine-iodine solution.

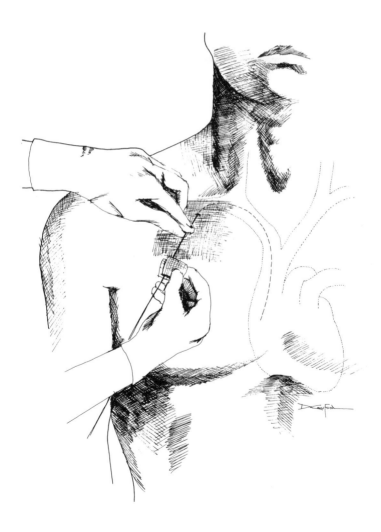

Figure 20: The new catheter is passed over the guidewire.

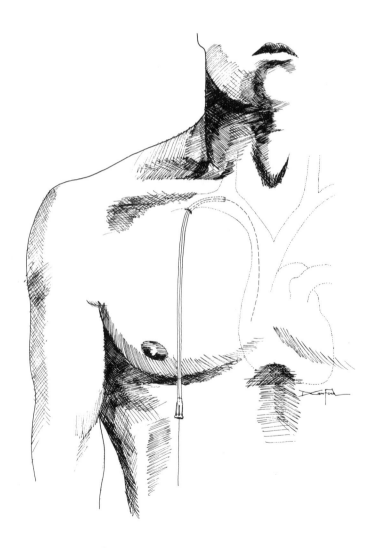

Figure 21: After removal of the guidewire, the newly placed catheter is aspirated to insure patency.

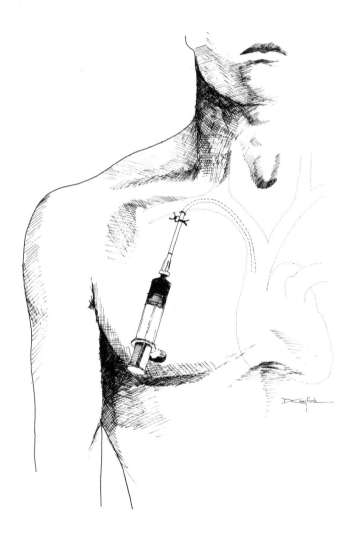

fluid and electrolyte status, tolerance to the glucose load, weekly assessment of metabolic parameters which may be altered with the nutritional program, and a catheter care program to insure freedom from infection or inadvertant contamination of the TPN line. To accomplish these tasks, the patient order form must include daily weights, strict intake and output with a separate listing for infused TPN, lipids, and other IV fluids which might include medications. Urine should be checked at 6-hour intervals for sugar and acetone. Electrolytes, glucose, and BUN should be analyzed daily until the patient is stable, and then on a periodic basis, i.e. Monday, Wednesday, and Friday. Assessment of the protime, albumin, magnesium, calcium, phosphate, and liver enzymes should be performed weekly to prevent the development of metabolic complications (Table III). Standing orders to start a peripheral IV of 10% glucose at the prescribed TPN rate should be provided for those occasions when the TPN line is inadvertantly discontinued or occluded. This measure will eliminate the hazards of hypoglycemia should the TPN line be discontinued or stopped for any prolonged period of time.

4/Subclavian Catheter Dressing Changes

In order to minimize catheter-related infections and complications, all staff involved with TPN care must follow stringent catheter care/dressing change guidelines. Using a standardized TPN Care Kit (Figure 22) eliminates the frustration of being unable to obtain the proper supplies and insures consistency in dressing care. The TPN Care Kit contains the following items:

1. Sterile gloves, size medium
2. 4x4 gauze sponges, 5 packages
3. 2x2 gauze sponges, 2 packages
4. 10x14 cm Opsite, 2 packages
5. Sterile extension tubing, 1 package
6. 10% iodine ointment, 1 package
7. Iodine ointment, 1 package
8. Face masks, 2 each

In addition, individuals responsible for dressing changes should carry a bottle of Freon TA and tincture of benzoin, 2-inch paper tape, and 2 iodine swabs.

All catheter dressings should be changed twice weekly,

Figure 22: The TPN Care Kit.

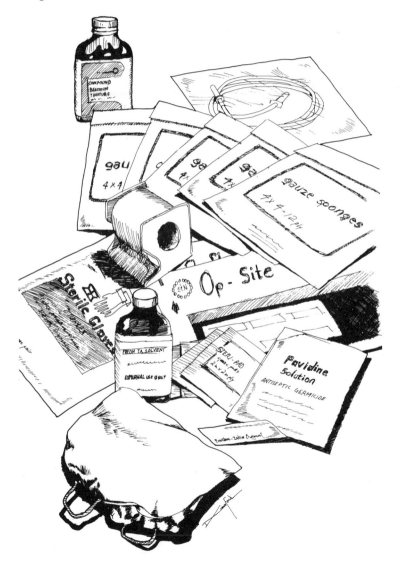

i.e. Monday and Thursday, and as needed according to the following protocol:

1. Assemble TPN Care Kit, Freon TA, tincture of benzoin, iodine swabs, and 2-inch paper tape in the patient's room.
2. Clear all materials off the bedside table and make sure the table top is clean.
3. WASH HANDS THOROUGHLY! (Figure 23).
4. Arrange supplies on clean table top near the area designated for the dressing change.
5. Don mask.
6. Open packages of 4x4's and place packages on the table so that none are touching. Be careful NOT TO TOUCH the insides of the packages. Open the packages of 2x2's by tearing in half and place opposite the 4x4's on a sterile package.
7. Holding container at least two inches from sponges, pour iodine solution over two packages of 4x4's (Figure 24).
8. Pour tincture of benzoin over the third 4x4 as in Step 7.
9. Squeeze one curl of iodine ointment into the middle of a 2x2 sponge.
10. Open Op-Site dressing.
11. Loosen and remove old dressing.
12. Place one iodine swab over the catheter hub and another over the flange of the extension tubing. Gently loosen connection, taking care NOT TO TOUCH the catheter with hands.
13. Remove extension tubing from its sterile package.
14. Crimp off (Z-fold) extension tubing at junction with the IV filter and disconnect (Figure 25).

15. Attach new extension tubing to filter and prime with IV solution. Keep extension tubing attached to the catheter crimped off during this entire portion of the procedure.
16. Ask the patient to take a deep breath and hold.
17. Using the iodine swabs, disconnect the old extension tubing from the catheter and quickly attach new extension tube, taking care not to touch the catheter hub with hands. Adjust extension tubing flange so that it lies flush with the skin.
18. Allow the patient to breathe normally.
19. Adjust the IV rate.
20. Pour Freon TA on remaining package of 4x4's, holding container 2 inches above the sponges.
21. Put on gloves.
22. Fold Freon TA 4x4's into 2x2 pad and gently, but firmly, cleanse the dressing area beginning at the catheter exit site and extending outward in a circular motion beyond the area to be redressed. Hold the catheter with the opposite hand to prevent dislodging (Figure 26). DO NOT wash the catheter or connections with Freon TA as it adversely affects properties of the catheter.
23. Cleanse twice with iodine 4x4's in the above fashion, each scrub lasting at least one minute and including the catheter and the first 3 inches of the extension tubing. Begin at the catheter site and cleanse outward beyond the area to be redressed.

24. Fold 2x2 gauze with iodine ointment directly over the catheter exit site. Fold one 2x2 and place under catheter-extension tubing connection. Place the remaining 2x2 gauzes longitudinally over the catheter cuff (Figure 27).

25. Fold 4x4 gauze in half and place lengthwise over catheter.

26. Fold tincture of benzoin 4x4 and wipe area surrounding gauze dressing, holding dressing with opposite hand to prevent displacement.

27. Remove gloves.

28. Place Op-Site adhesive over gauze dressing, extending at least 1/2 inch on each side, then press firmly from the bottom up to insure adhesion (Figure 28).

29. Coil exposed tubing loosely over the dressing and secure with two 3-inch strips of paper tape.

30. Date and sign dressing.

Figure 23: WASH HANDS THOROUGHLY!

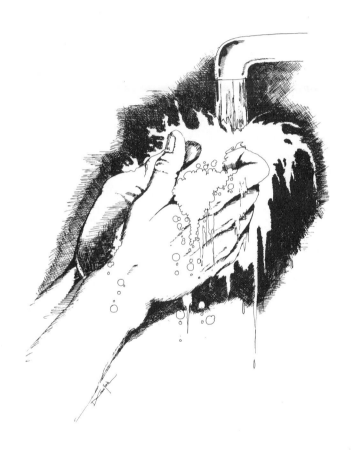

Figure 24: Proper layout of 4x4's and 2x2's on table top as they are prepped with povidine solution.

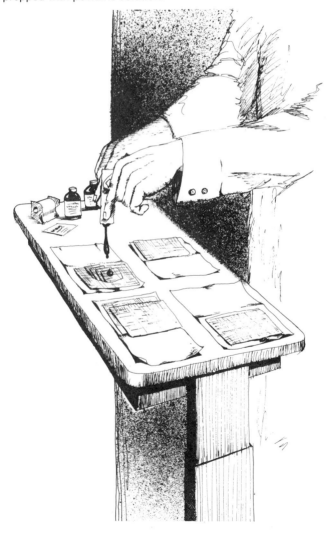

Figure 25: Crimping off extension tubing at junction with the IV filter.

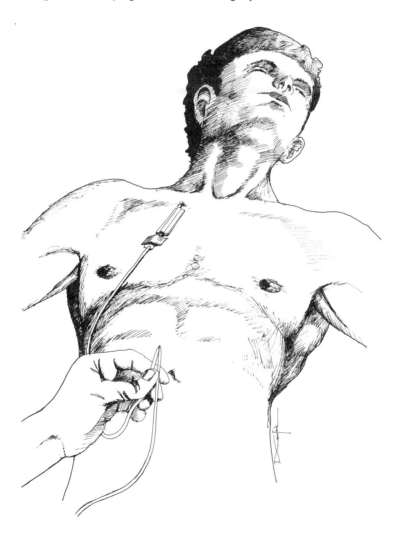

Figure 26: Holding the catheter to prevent dislodging, the catheter exit site is cleansed in a circular motion extending outward beyond the area to be redressed.

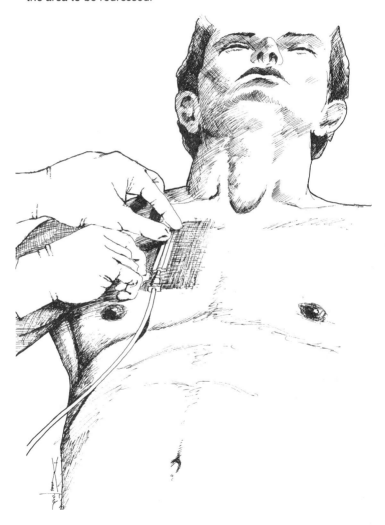

Figure 27: Placement of 2x2 gauze sponges over the catheter exit site, under the catheter-extension tubing connection and longitudinally over the catheter cuff.

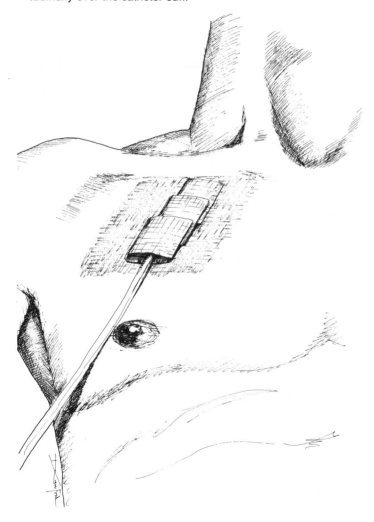

Figure 28: Op-Site adhesive over gauze dressing extending at least 1/2 inch on each side. Green strips may be removed after adhesion is insured.

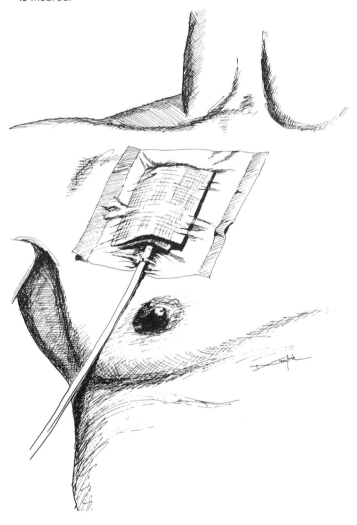

5/Selection of Solutions

To select the proper solution that will provide the necessary calories and protein, some basic information is required to calculate the availability of these substrates in solution.

Non-Nitrogen Calories

Caloric requirements should be provided from a non-nitrogen source. Available non-nitrogen energy substrates are glucose, glycerol, and lipid. Protein, the only nitrogen source, should be excluded from any caloric calculations. Although glucose commonly provides 4 calories per gram of substrate, the hydrous form of glucose available in IV solutions provides only 3.4 calories of energy to the patient. Therefore, 500 ml of 50% glucose, which contains 250 grams of glucose, would provide 850 calories. These calculations are based on the fact that 50% glucose provides 50 grams of glucose per 100 cc of solution; thus, 500 ml would provide 250 grams of glucose, and 250 x 3.4 = 850 calories.

Lipids generate 9 calories per gram of substrate; thus 500 ml of 10% lipid would provide 450 calories. However, because lipids are provided as an emulsion without osmolarity, 25 grams of 5% glycerol have been added to the solution to provide a suitable osmolarity. Glycerol is metabolized similar to glucose and provides 4 calories per gram of substrate. Thus, 100 additional calories from glycerol are provided in the 500 ml of 10% lipid solution. The combination of lipid and glycerol total 550 calories per 500 ml, or 1.1 (non-nitrogen) calories per ml solution.

Nitrogen Concentrations

Proteins provide the nitrogen source necessary for protein synthesis. Although grams of protein are commonly calculated in the nutritional support plan, grams of nitrogen are occasionally used as an expression of the amount of protein being provided. The conversion factor of protein to nitrogen is important and should be well understood. Nitrogen comprises approximately 16% of the total weight of all proteins. Calculating grams of nitrogen from protein is achieved by dividing the grams of protein by 6.25. This calculation will determine the grams of nitrogen available in a protein solution. Using the standard 500 ml of 8.5% amino acid solution, calculations to determine grams of nitrogen follow: 8.5% indicates 8.5 grams of amino acid per 100 ml of solution; 500 ml would then provide 42.5 grams of protein equivalent amino acid in the solution. Dividing 42.5 grams by 6.25 determines that 6.8 grams of nitrogen are available in 500 ml of 8.5% amino acid solution.

Calorie/Nitrogen Ratio

Calorie to nitrogen ratios are frequently referred to in nutrition literature. This ratio is determined by dividing the total *non-nitrogen calories* available by the grams of nitrogen being provided. A TPN solution composed of 500 ml of 50% dextrose and 500 ml of 8.5% amino acid solution would have the following calorie to nitrogen ratio: 850 calories/6.8 grams nitrogen = 125/1 ratio of non-nitrogen calories to grams of nitrogen. The usual ratio of non-nitrogen calories to nitrogen is in the range of 150-300/1. In the stressed or septic patient, a lower ratio of 125/1 may be more appropriate since some of the protein provided may be utilized as an energy substrate in pathways that are available or selectively preferred in stressed patients.

Selection of the Specific Solution

Standard solutions of TPN provide many advantages to an active nutrition support service. Although they do not provide the individual variances needed for specific patients, development of a standard solution protocol will streamline the nutritional support program and will prove to be safe and cost-effective when used appropriately. Standard solutions composed of an appropriate blend of glucose, proteins, electrolytes, vitamins, and trace minerals insure that all nutritional elements are provided to the patient, irrespective of the clinician's expertise in formulating a TPN prescription. Ordering TPN with standard solution designations, i.e. TPN Solution A, provides an easily recognizable physician order which the pharmacist can interpret without numerous calls for clarification. Using standard TPN solutions, the pharmacist can estimate the number of solutions needed and prepare them prior to receiving specific orders. At Butterworth Hospital, standard solutions are designated by capital letters and are ordered as TPN Solution A, B, E,

F, or D at the physician's discretion. The formulations of each standard solution are available on each floor and in the TPN protocol. Although each standard solution is prepared to meet the usual patient requirements, each TPN solution can be adjusted to meet individual needs. This can be accomplished with little effort, yet maintains the clarity in orders and the efficiency of the system.

TPN Solution A

Solution A is prepared from 500 ml of 50% glucose and 500 ml of 8.5% amino acid solution with electrolytes; 4.5 mEq of calcium gluconate is added to the blended solution (Table IV). 1000 ml of Solution A provides 850 non-protein calories from glucose, 42.5 grams of amino acid (protein) which yields 6.8 grams of nitrogen, giving a 125/1 non-protein calorie to nitrogen ratio. Electrolytes provided in one liter of this solution are 35 mEq sodium, 30 mEq potassium, 5 mEq magnesium, and 4.5 mEq calcium. Anions are provided as 35 mEq chloride, 30 mEq phosphate, and 65 mEq acetate.

TPN Solution A is the most common TPN solution used at Butterworth Hospital and nationwide. Although higher quantities of protein (amino acid) are provided than may be needed for all patients, most seem to utilize the protein effectively, if normal renal function prevails. The higher protein concentration is particularly beneficial in the stressed or septic patient who may preferentially be utilizing proteins as an energy source due to altered metabolic states. Our studies regarding energy substrate utilization have indicated that proteins contribute 20-25% of the energy source and, in some patients, greater amounts of protein are selectively utilized as the energy substrate, irrespective of the amount of non-protein calories being provided. Higher protein concentrations in the TPN solution are especially desirable when lower energy requirements restrict the volume of TPN being infused. Conversely, in patients with impaired renal function due to chronic disease, it may be advisable to select a TPN solution providing lower concentrations of protein.

TPN Solution B

Solution B has the same nutrient composition as A, however all electrolytes are deleted except for a necessary 26 mEq of acetate and 17 mEq of chloride used in the amino acid preparation (Table V). The advantages of an electrolyte-depleted solution are particularly important in the management of patients with electrolyte imbalances or acid-base disorders. This is especially true for those patients with hypercalcemia, hyperkalemia, or hypernatremic states in which elimination of the cation from the infusion is essential. Elimination of all sodium has been helpful in managing patients with fluid retention and dilutional hyponatremia commonly found with hepatic failure or ascites due to tumor. The ability to modify the electrolyte pattern also helps patients with acid-base disorders. Metabolic alkalosis frequently will respond well to reconstituting the electrolyte profile using chloride as the anion in all added electrolytes, i.e. 35 mEq NaCl, 30 mEq KCl, and 5 mEq CaCl. Adjusting the solution in such a manner can provide up to an additional 50 mEq of chloride in the TPN solution without altering the cation concentrations.

TPN Solutions E and F

The protein concentration in Solutions E and F (5.5% amino acid) is the only major difference from TPN solutions A and B. A liter of either E or F solution will provide 27.5 grams of amino acid (protein). Solution E contains the pre-mixed electrolytes similar to the pattern described for Solution A, while the F Solution contains proteins and calories without any significant electrolyte content (Tables VI and VII). The nitrogen content in this solution is calculated as follows: 500 ml x 5.5% = 27.5 grams of amino acid divided by 6.25 = 4.4 grams of nitrogen. Dividing the grams of nitrogen into the 850 calories provided by the 500 ml of glucose gives a calorie to nitrogen ratio of 193/1. This higher calorie to nitrogen ratio falls within the physiologic parameters for a non-stressed adult person, thus, this solution may be appropriate for the hospitalized patient who does not require the higher protein concentrations for wound healing or other reparative processes.

The lower protein concentration in these solutions may be suitable for patients with marginal renal or hepatic function. The E or F Solution would be the solutions of choice for a patient with an elevated BUN and a stable, but mildly elevated, creatinine. Patients with jaundice or evidence of liver impairment, i.e. elevated liver function tests or cirrhosis, may not tolerate the higher protein concentrations found in Solutions A and B, but may do well with Solution F. This is particularly relevant when infusing TPN at rates of 2.5-3 liters per day. The selective utilization of branched chain amino acids by these patients and their limited ability to convert ammonium to urea gives rise to serious concern for the amount of protein infused daily.

TPN Solution D (Surgery Solution)

Solution D was developed as a TPN solution to be used during the perioperative period when the stress of operative trauma could induce great fluctuations in the serum glucose. The D Solution is composed of 500 ml 8.5% amino acid solution without electrolytes and 500 ml of 20% glucose (Table VIII). The amino acids and minimal glucose concentrations provide the protein sparing desired and reduce the hazards of hyperglycemia caused by the release of epinephrine, glucocorticosteroid, and glucagon during and immediately after the operation. It also prevents the development of hypoglycemia which could occur if the standard TPN solutions were discontinued for a prolonged operative period. The omission of electrolytes in TPN Solution D eliminates the hazards of hyperkalemia in the immediate post-operative period and provides a constant fluid volume (50 ml/hour) which can be used as a part of the fluid replacement during and immediately after the operation.

Solution D should be started at 50 ml per hour 6 hours prior to the anticipated surgery and continued at this rate for the first 24 hours post-operatively. A standard TPN solution such as Solution A or E may be resumed on the first post-op day at 50 cc per hour and gradually increased in rate to meet the patient's requirements. Maintaining a TPN solution during surgery has the added advantage of alerting the anesthesiologist and the surgery team that the central venous line is a TPN line which should not be used for infusion of drugs or blood products unless an absolute emergency arises.

TPN Solution S-1

This solution was developed to meet the metabolic needs of patients in renal failure. Simplicity and cost effective issues also were a concern in the evolution of this product. The nutritional requirements for a patient with oliguric renal failure must be modified considerably to meet the special metabolic limitations. Although the caloric requirements are essentially unaltered from the normal patient, tolerance to protein and nitrogen is drastically reduced. In addition, fluid volumes must be markedly limited unless the patient is on a regular dialysis program. Careful monitoring of glucose, potassium, and magnesium in addition to the renal function parameters is especially important in this group of patients. The S-1 Solution, composed of 125 ml of 8.5% amino acid solution without electrolytes and 500 ml 50% dextrose, provides 10.6 grams of amino acids with 1.7 grams of nitrogen and 850 non-nitrogen calories (Table IX). The calorie to nitrogen ratio of 500/1 provides a high caloric intake with very limited quantities of protein (nitrogen). The cost of materials (amino acids and glucose) to produce this solution is significantly less than for a standard TPN solution and drastically cheaper than commercially available renal failure solutions.

The historical development of the present concepts of amino acid synthesis and utilization in the renal failure patient plays a major role in the nutrition support program offered. The action of bacterial urease on urea in the gut to produce amino radicles sets the stage for the amination of alpha-keto analogues in the intestinal circulation. This metabolic pathway is capable of producing non-essential amino acids. Essential amino acids, which cannot be synthesized through this same process, are necessary for protein synthesis. The actualization of this concept led to the development of essential amino acid solutions in the treatment of renal failure. A closer review of the pioneering studies by Giordano[23] found that the limited quantities of protein used in their dietary programs were not essential amino acids, but high-quality proteins, i.e. egg albumin. The ratio of non-nitrogen calories to grams of nitrogen approached 500/1.

On the basis of this information, the present S-1 solution was developed utilizing a limited quantity of quality protein which is present in the standard TPN product. The high caloric density and the limited volume achieve the objectives required in the treatment of oliguric renal failure. The addition of sodium, potassium and magnesium must be monitored carefully. Additional potassium is usually required once nutritional support is initiated, and hyperglycemia is common with serum glucose levels of 200-300 mg/dl. Significant amounts of added insulin may be required to maintain these concentrations. Sodium is added only as deemed necessary since the normal renal excretory mechanisms no longer prevail. The effectiveness of this solution in the treatment of oliguric renal failure is difficult to determine due to the limited clinical usage of such solutions. However, in the past seven years, this solution has been used without complication in our institution. The recent introduction of 20% lipid offers great advantages in that a highly dense caloric fluid is now available without the disadvantages associated with previously required concentrated glucose solutions.

Nutritional support orders for a patient with oliguric renal failure with fluid restrictions can be developed from the TPN S-1 Solution and 20% lipid in the following manner: TPN Solution S-1 at an infusion rate of 25ml/hour provides 600 ml of fluid, 800 calories, 10 grams of protein, and 1.5 grams of nitrogen. Infusing 20% lipid at 5 ml per hour adds an additional 120 ml of fluid and 240 calories. Thus, the combined TPN solution and lipids will provide 1040 calories, 10 grams of protein, and a total volume of 720 ml of fluid. This combination of non-nitrogen caloric sources with limited amounts of protein provides a calorie to nitrogen ratio of 690:1.

High output renal failure is more common than oliguric renal failure and can be equally challenging to treat. Urine volumes and specific gravity must be monitored closely, and urine and serum electrolytes, creatinine, and osmolarity must be checked regularly to quantitate the replacement of solutions. Volume replacement is calculated carefully at 12-hour intervals or more frequently if dramatic urine volume changes are occurring. Nutritional requirements of non-nitrogen calories, protein, vitamins, and electrolytes are determined and distributed equally in the fluids infused throughout the day. The use of 3-liter bags has helped immeasurably in providing the necessary fluids and nutritional elements on a continuous basis throughout a 24-hour period.

TPN Solution S-2

This special solution is a step up in proteins from the S-1 Solution. TPN S-2 is composed of 500 ml of 50% glucose and 250 ml of 8.5% amino acids without electrolytes (Table X). This 750 ml of fluid provides 21.25 grams of protein (3.4 grams of nitrogen) and 850 calories, giving a calorie to nitrogen ratio of 250/1. Again, electrolytes must be added as needed. This solution is indicated for those patients who have begun to show improvement on the S-1 renal failure solution, usually signalled by a declining BUN and an increasing urine output. Under these circumstances, every effort should be made to increase the protein load to tolerance in an effort to insure adequate protein replacement for the reparative process and restoration of nutritional deficiencies. This solution is especially useful when the TPN solution is blended with lipids. The combined non-nitrogen calories from glucose and lipid will require higher protein concentrations to achieve the calorie to nitrogen ratio desired.

6/ Other TPN Solutions

TPN Formula for Pulmonary Failure

The pulmonary failure patient on ventilatory support is becoming an ever-increasing nutritional management problem. These patients classically are markedly malnourished with depleted body fat stores and a reduction of lean body mass. Frequently, a super-imposed pulmonary infection on an already incapacitating chronic obstructive pulmonary disease leads to further depletion of the energy stores. Visceral proteins are particularly vulnerable to this acute catabolic process. Nutritional support is indicated, but frequently omitted due to the marked restriction of fluid intake and the need for multiple IV medications.[24] Establishing a nutritional support program for this type of patient is a major challenge requiring close communication with the attending physicians. The objectives are to provide 1.0 grams of protein per kilogram and to meet the energy requirements with a balanced energy source of fat and carbohydrate. The limitation of glucose as an energy source is necessary to keep the CO_2 generation at acceptable levels.[25] A limited fluid volume is also essential. These objectives can be accomplished with a specially prepared solution of 500 ml 8.5% amino acid which provides 42.5 grams of protein (amino acids), and 350 ml of 70% glucose which contributes 245 grams of glucose and 833 calories (Table XI). The total 850 ml of solution can be infused in 24 hours at a rate of 35 ml per hour; 20% lipid infused at 15 ml per hour directly into the TPN line provides an additional 720 calories and 360 ml of fluid. Using this combined lipid/70% glucose formula, 1550 calories and 42.5 grams of protein can be provided to the patient at a total IV rate of 50 ml per hour, or 1.2 liters per day. This mix provides approximately 50% of the non-nitrogen calories from fat and a similar amount from carbohydrate. Most patients on a fluid-restricted program and ventilator tolerate this parenteral program well without evidence of fluid accumulation, and it is sufficiently volume-concentrated to allow the infusion of antibiotics and bronchodilators in minimal dilutions without risk of fluid overload. The equal caloric contribution from fat and carbohydrate limits the CO_2 generation while providing sufficient carbohydrate calories for basal metabolic function.

TPN Solutions for Fluid Overload Syndromes

Patients with excessive fluid retention as manifested by marked peripheral edema, ascites, pleural effusion, or anasarca, usually represent chronic disease processes such as hepatic cirrhosis, ovarian carcinoma, and other neoplasms with peritoneal implantation. Congestive heart failure resulting from constrictive pericarditis or cardiac insufficiency can also cause these conditions. The serum sodium in this group of patients is usually low (120-135 mEq/liter) and, in chronic states, may be as low as 115-120 mEq per liter. The low serum sodium levels are frequently interpreted as a total body sodium deficit, when in reality, the total body sodium is usually above normal. The combined influences of aldosterone and ADH released as a result of low intravascular volumes due to capillary leak result in excessive sodium and fluid retention.

The management objectives for these patients are to provide the necessary energy requirements to fuel the sodium pump and other transport systems, restrict volume, limit sodium intake, and provide appropriate protein and vitamin supplementation. These measures when applied with appropriate management of the underlying disease process and judicious use of diuretics (furosemide) can produce dramatic results within 7-10 days. A typical solution for a patient with these problems would be compounded as follows: 500 ml 8.5% amino acid solution without electrolytes and 500 ml 70% glucose solution. One liter of this solution would provide 1200 non-protein calories and 42.5 grams of amino acid (Table XII). Thirty mEq KCl, 8 mEq $MgSO_4$, and 4.5 mEq calcium are added initially and adjusted according to the patient's requirements. Infusing this solution at 50 ml per hour (1.2 liters/24 hours) provides 1500 calories and 50 grams of protein. All other medications are given in minimal dilutions, IV push, or IM in an effort to maintain the volume-restriction program, and patients are kept NPO or fluid-restricted. MVI 12 and trace minerals are added to each liter of solution to insure that total nutritional needs are being met. A minimum effective dose of furosemide (Lasix) is given IV push every 6-8 hours in an effort to induce a mild continuous diuresis of the retained fluid.

The over-aggressive use of diuretics may induce a temporary hypotension which usually responds to 500 ml of isotonic solution. The use of albumin to effect an increased intravascular oncotic pressure may provide temporary benefits; however, in the presence of capillary leak, albumin readily passes into the interstitial spaces where it further aggravates the fluid retention problems. Even in those conditions where the albumin may be as low as 1.5 grams/dl, we have been able to effectively manage these patients without the infusion of exogenous albumin.

7/All in One TPN Solution

The development of large volume, flexible plastic IV fluid bags, and the documented stability of carbohydrates, lipids, proteins, electrolytes, trace minerals and vitamins for prolonged periods of time has permitted the development of a comprehensive 24-hour nutritional formula termed "All in one TPN solution." This system offers several advantages for the stable patient requiring TPN.

1. A blended formula of all required nutrients can be infused constantly throughout a 24-hour period.
2. An individualized "nutritional" program is developed for each patient.
3. Nursing requirements are reduced in that one bag is hung and infused continuously over a 24-hour period.
4. Risk of contaminating a TPN infusion line is reduced, as only one bag is connected to the central line during each 24-hour period.

Writing the Order

Starting a patient on the "all in one system" requires thorough assessment of the patient, a determination of the nutritional need, and a thoughtful patient management plan, as noted on the metabolic nutritional support service consultation form (See Figures 1, 29). In the all in one TPN solution, non-protein calories can be provided as a blend of carbohydrates and fats similar to a normal diet (i.e., 60–70% carbohydrate and 30–40% fat). Proteins are provided as amino acid solutions (usually 1 to 1½ grams per kilogram). Appropriate electrolytes, trace minerals and vitamins are added to provide a complete nutritional formula.

Example

A six foot male patient, formerly weighing 180 lbs., has lost 20 lbs. in the past six weeks and will require IV nutrition prior to a planned operation. His ideal weight is 178 lbs. (80 kilograms), and the nutrition plan will be based on the ideal weight. The caloric requirement (non-protein) is 2,000 calories per 24-hour period. 500 ml of 10% lipid will provide 550 calories. The remaining 1,400 calories could be provided by 410 grams of glucose. Thus, an all in one TPN order could be individualized to meet this patient's need by the following prescription:

500 ml	10% lipid	=	550 calories
800 ml	50% glucose	=	1400 calories
		=	1950 total non-protein calories
1000 ml	8.5% amino acid	=	85 grams of protein

Trace minerals and vitamins would be added using standard requirements and adjusted daily until normal serum electrolyte levels are established. Infusion of the all in one solution at 95 ccs per hour would use the entire TPN formula within a 24-hour period.

Limitations

The disadvantages of the all in one solution are primarily limited to the loss of flexibility in changing solutions without destroying large volumes of TPN. Thus, it is essential that patients be stabilized before placing them into an all in one TPN solution. Experience with this TPN method has found that the prescribed solution can be initiated at the desired rate without the need to start at a lowered rate of delivery. It is advisable to modify the solution and taper off slowly as the patient resumes normal alimentation.

Figure 29: All in One TPN Solution Order Form.

☐ **Non-Standard Central Solution**
Base Solution:

Dextrose	Amino Acids	Lipids
DEX 20% _____ml	A.A. 8.5%* _____ml	Lipids 10% _____ml
DEX 50% _____ml	(1.43gm N/100ml)	(1.1Kcal per ml)
DEX 70% _____ml	A.A. 10%* _____ml	Lipids 20% _____ml
DEX ____% _____ml	(1.53gm N/100ml)	(2.0Kcal per ml)
(provides 3.4Kcal	*contains Phosphate 10mm/L	
per gm of dextrose)	(hepatic and renal solutions	
	available upon request)	

sterile water q.s. _____ml

E-LYTE ADDITIVES:

NaCL	_____ meq	
Na Acetate	_____ meq	
Na Phosphate	_____ meq (Na)	(3mm Phos per 4 meq Na)
KCL	_____ meq	
K Acetate	_____ meq	
K Phosphate	_____ meq (K)	(3mm Phos per 4.4 meq K)
Ca Gluconate	_____ meq	
Mg Sulfate	_____ meq	

MISC. ADDITIVES:

_____ MVI   1 vial daily

_____ Trace Minerals 1ml/daily
(Zn 5mg, Cu 1 mg, Mn 0.5mg, Cr 10mcg)

Heparin _____ units

Reg. Insulin _____ units

Vitamin K _____ mg/Freq. _____

Misc. _____
_____
_____

RATE: _____ ml/hr.

Adult Daily Parenteral Requirements	
Na	50-250 meq
K	30-200 meq
Cl	50-250 meq
Ca	10-20 meq
Mg	10-30 meq
Phos	10-40 mm

Physician's Signature: _____ Date: _____

8/Additives and Adjustments to TPN Solutions

Vitamins and Trace Minerals

A well balanced vitamin preparation (MVI 12) and 1 cc of a standard trace mineral preparation containing 4 mg zinc, 1 mg copper, 0.5 mg manganese, and 10 mcg chromium are added to one bag of TPN solution per day (Tables XIII and XIV). In our system, MIV 12 and the trace minerals will be added when designated on the order form as standard additives. Vitamin K and Vitamin B_{12} and extra zinc should be considered for patients with GI diseases.

Patients with advanced malnutrition due to prolonged starvation or extreme stress, i.e. sepsis, steroids, or chemotherapy, can be assumed to have major vitamin and trace mineral deficiencies. It has been our practice to provide standard additives (MVI 12 and trace minerals) to each bag of TPN for the first 3-5 days. Thus, patients receiving 2-3 liters of TPN per day will receive excess micronutrients which may be necessary for their depleted state. Documenting vitamin deficiencies poses difficulties since analysis of vitamins other than folic acid and

B_{12} is not commonly available. These tests are usually expensive, and serum analysis may not reflect cellular levels. Long-term overdosing with vitamins A and D may create clinical problems. Thus, continued overdosing with standard additives may prove harmful, especially in the long-term home care patients. Vitamin B_{12} is now present in the newly formulated MVI 12; however, in patients started on TPN with long-standing disease processes involving the stomach or terminal ileum, i.e. lymphoma, Crohn's disease, or short bowel syndrome, 1000 units of vitamin B_{12} should be administered IM to replenish existing deficiencies.

Vitamin K is not included in the vitamin preparation and may be necessary. Prolongation of the prothrombin time or partial thromboplastin time will signal a deficiency in vitamin K which is needed in the synthesis of prothrombin, a coagulation factor. This vitamin deficiency, although rare, does occur with some regularity in TPN patients. The natural presence of vitamin K in foods and the endogenous synthesis of vitamin K by intestinal flora may be altered by poor oral intake and the long-term use of oral antibiotics. Thus, elderly or chronically ill patients with limited oral intake due to obstruction or anorexia may be at great risk for vitamin K deficiencies, especially when placed on long-standing oral antibiotic therapy. Vitamin K supplementation can be provided on a regular basis by adding small amounts to one bag of TPN daily. Another alternative calls for monitoring TPN patients for vitamin K deficiencies by performing a PT or PTT on a weekly basis. Those patients with a prolongation of the protime by one second or prolongation of the PTT are given 10 mg of vitamin K in the next bag of TPN, and the protime is rechecked. This method has proven to be cost-effective, as the daily addition of vitamin K is expensive and may not be necessary for all patients. No adverse reactions have been noted with the addition of vitamin K to TPN solutions, even though problems have been described when the drug is given IV. [26,27]

Additional zinc may be required for those patients having excessive GI losses. Patients with high output ileostomies or prolonged NG suction are routinely given 4-12 mg of zinc in the daily TPN in addition to the usual trace minerals. Serum zinc levels are monitored weekly on all TPN patients and any noted deficiency is appropriately treated.

Glucose Concentrations in Standard TPN Solutions

Although the standard TPN solution is compounded with 50% glucose, alterations in the glucose concentration can be initiated by listing the standard solution and following this designation with a change in the glucose percentage in parentheses, i.e. Standard Solution A (D30). This simplistic method of designating changes in the glucose concentration is especially time-saving for the clinician and is equally beneficial to the pharmacist preparing the solution who, in the past, frequently was confronted with long, drawn-out descriptions of the solution that were open to great error.

Hyperglycemia

Hyperglycemia, noted in the diabetic or stressed, insulin-resistant patient, is usually managed with the addition of regular insulin to the TPN bag or bottle. Although a small quantity of insulin may adhere to the container, sufficient insulin is infused to effect the desired changes in blood glucose or glycosuria. The objective of a well-monitored system is to maintain the blood glucose between 100-200 mg/dl. Patients noted to spill 3+ or 4+ glucose in the urine should have immediate blood sugars drawn. Patients with blood sugars above 200 mg/dl are placed on blood sugar analyses every 6 hours until satisfactory control is achieved. Blood sugars above 200 are treated by adding 1 unit of regular insulin per 100 cc of solution remaining in the bag, and all subsequent bags of TPN solution have 10 additional units of regular insulin added. Additional regular insulin is added, based on the results of 6 hour blood sugars, up to a maximum of 100 units per liter. Once the maximum insulin level is reached, if the hyperglycemia (above 200 mg/dl) persists, the glucose concentration in the TPN solution should be reduced. This is usually achieved by reducing the concentration to 30% written as follows: TPN Solution A (D30). Lipids may be needed to augment the non-nitrogen caloric source under these circumstances. The following case is presented as an example:

TPN Solution A is started on Mr. X at 50 ml per hour at 8:00 a.m. Glycosuria of 3+ is noted at 10:00 a.m., and a blood sugar is drawn which is reported at 350 mg/dl. Nine hundred ml of TPN solution remains in the bag, and 9 units of regular insulin is added. Six hours later (4:00 p.m.), a repeat blood sugar of 300 mg/dl is obtained. Six hundred ml of the first liter of TPN is hanging, and an additional 6 units of regular insulin is added. Orders are written so that liter #2 will contain 20 units of regular insulin. A blood glucose drawn at 10:00 p.m. reports a blood sugar of 275 mg/dl. In liter #1, 300 ml of TPN remains. Three additional units of regular insulin are added to bag #1, and an order is written so that liter #2 will be formulated with 30 units of regular insulin. Six hours later, liter #2 with 30 units of regular insulin is hanging, and the blood sugar is reported at 175 mg/dl. All subsequent liters of TPN will be ordered with 30 units of regular insulin, and daily blood sugars will be obtained to insure blood glucose levels above 100 but below 200 mg/dl.

Improvement in the clinical problem is usually associated with an improvement in insulin resistance, and when this occurs, blood sugars may drop below 100. The insulin level should be reduced by 10 units in the next liter of TPN solution which is hung as soon as possible. Blood glucose levels should be checked at 6-12 hour intervals and appropriate reductions in insulin implemented. When high levels of insulin are used in the TPN solution and the stress response is resolving, it is advisable to draw blood sugars one hour prior to hanging each new liter and adjust the insulin dosage at that time.

Patients who persist to have glycosuria in spite of acceptable blood glucose levels may have a good response with the addition of ten units of regular insulin to the bag of solution. Frequently this added insulin will elevate the renal threshold for glucose such that glycosuria no longer occurs. Commonly, within 2-3 days, the insulin can be discontinued without further occurrence of glycosuria.

Hypokalemia

The infusion of high quantities of glucose and the restoration of intracellular enzyme systems is commonly associated with large shifts of potassium intracellularly. Potassium, up to 200 mEq or more, may be required daily to restore the intracellular potassium deficits. Potassium can be added to the TPN solution as potassium chloride, potassium acetate, or potassium phosphate. The choice of anion will depend upon the acid-base status and/or the identification of a phosphate deficiency. A low serum potassium in association with normal serum bicarbonate levels should be replaced as potassium chloride. A bicarbonate level below 20 suggests acidosis, and it may be advisable to add potassium as K acetate. A phosphate level below 2.5 in association with a low potassium level is an indication for potassium phosphate replacement. Because of the variable equilibrium between potassium and hydrogen ion with the bivalent phosphate anion, it is best to order K phosphate in terms of millimoles of phosphate and to check with the pharmacist to determine the potassium concentration in the additive. Usually, a 2 to 3 relationship of phosphate to potassium is available in the solution; thus, 10 millimoles of phosphate will deliver 15 mEq of potassium.

Guides for estimating the quantity of potassium replacement required are fraught with errors due to the large quantity of intracellular potassium (4200 mEq in a 70 Kg male) and the minimal concentrations available as serum potassium (14 mEq in a 70 Kg male). A serum potassium of 3.5 mEq/L could represent only minimal potassium deficiencies in a relatively healthy individual, whereas the same reading in a chronically ill patient receiving daily diuretics would likely indicate a major potassium deficit. Thus, potassium replacement requires knowledge of the patient and good clinical assessment skills in addition to reliable laboratory tests. When in doubt, one should add reasonable amounts of potassium

(20-30 mEq/liter) and reassess the serum potassium in a specific time period, i.e. 6-8 hours.

Hypocalcemia

Calcium levels below 8.5 mg/dl are noted quite frequently in the malnourished patient with visceral protein deficiencies (adult kwashiorkor). Although calcium replacement may be necessary, adjustments must be made in relation to the serum albumin. A deficit of one gram of albumin will account for an associated reduction in the serum calcium of 0.8 mg/dl. Thus, a patient with a serum albumin of 2.5 grams and a serum calcium of 8 mEq would fall within the normal range with the adjustment of an added 0.8 mg of calcium for the one gram of albumin needed to bring the albumin to normal levels. An additional 4.5 mEq of calcium as gluconate might be acceptable, but would not be necessary.

Magnesium Replacement

Patients with a magnesium below 1.5 mg/dl should have additional magnesium sulfate added to TPN solution. Magnesium is available in multiples of 4 mEq; thus a patient with a serum magnesium of 1.2 should receive an additional 8 mEq of magnesium in each liter of TPN solution until a repeat serum magnesium falls within the normal range. At that point, the 5 mEq of magnesium included in TPN Solution A and E will suffice.

Phosphate Additives

Phosphate is available in association with sodium or potassium cations. Although hypophosphatemia was a common problem with the early amino acid solutions, present solutions provide adequate amounts of phosphate for most patients. Identification of a serum phosphate below 2.5 mg% is an indication for the addition of potassium or sodium phosphate to assure adequate quantities of this ion to permit the phosphorylation of glucose needed to metabolize glucose into an energy source. It should be remembered that phosphate should be ordered in millimoles to eliminate the confusion associated with ordering milliequivalents of a bivalent anion in equilibrium with two cation molecules.

Acid-Base Disorders

TPN patients requiring nutritional support frequently have associated acid-base problems. Commonly, the acid-base imbalance exists prior to starting TPN. However, the TPN solutions and treatment for the underlying problems, i.e. NG suction for gastric or intestinal obstruction or ventilators and Lasix, can also give rise to major acid-base problems.

Metabolic acidosis is commonly associated with hypoperfusion and volume deficits. A serum bicarbonate less than 24 mEq/liter may be used to identify and treat metabolic acidosis, providing a primary respiratory problem can be ruled out. Arterial blood gases are indicated initially to establish a diagnosis, but may not be necessary for continued management of the problem. Sodium bicarbonate, the common therapy for metabolic acidosis, cannot be used in TPN solutions due to precipitation caused by the calcium and magnesium ions. Acetate, which is metabolized to bicarbonate in the liver, can be added in large quantities without risk of precipitation. Estimates of the acetate required to correct the metabolic acidosis may be determined from the following formula: body weight (Kg) x 0.3 x (25 minus the serum bicarbonate). The acetate is available as the sodium or potassium salt. The required amount should be given in the TPN solutions over a 24 hour period. Repeat electrolytes the following morning are needed to determine the effectiveness of the therapy and to recalculate the acetate requirements for the following 24 hours should a deficit persist.

Metabolic alkalosis is becoming an increasingly common problem in hospitalized patients. This is caused by the large hydrochloric acid losses associated with an NG tube or vomiting, frequent use of potent diuretics (furosemide), and the mineral corticoid effects of steroids. Metabolic alkalosis is identified from the serum electrolytes as a bicarbonate level above 28 mEq. The base excess can be calculated as follows: total body weight (Kg) x 0.3 x (serum bicarbonate minus 27). Replacement of the calculated base excess and fluid deficits with normal saline and added KCl is the standard therapy. Patients refractory to standard treatment and those with organ failure, i.e. renal, hepatic, or pulmonary failure, may require hydrochloric acid to correct the base excess. HCl (2 mEq/ml) can be prepared in the hospital pharmacy by appropriate dilution and filtering of concentrated HCl solutions. Our experience with hydrochloric acid in TPN has proven its safety and effectiveness when added to solutions containing amino acids. The amino acids provide an effective buffer, and infusion through a central line eliminates the risks associated with peripheral administration. Up to 1600 mEq of HCl have been given to one patient over a 5-day period without complication.[28]

Iron

Iron deficiency anemia is commonly identified in the malnourished patient. The anemia may occur as a result of inadequate oral intake of iron-containing foods, or faulty absorptive mechanisms. Gross or occult blood loss from chronic inflammatory bowel disease, carcinoma, or the complications of recent surgery may have precipitated the problem. Transfusions of red blood cells may not be necessary or desired if the patient's erythropoetic system can be stimulated to produce its own red cells. Restoring the nutritional status and repleting the iron stores should be considered if the clinical condition does not require immediate transfusion.

Oral iron is frequently poorly tolerated, especially in patients with GI disorders. The intramuscular injection of iron is painful, may cause discoloration of the skin, and may be a stimulus for the development of sarcoma. The use of parenteral iron as an IV bolus has been reported with good success. However, allergic reactions, especially in patients with collagen disorders, have deterred from its widespread acceptance. Iron therapy in the severely malnourished patient also has been associated with an increased incidence of sepsis, even though iron is necessary for a properly functioning immune system.

The Nutrition Support Service at Butterworth Hospital has used an iron-dextran solution (Imferon) as an additive to TPN solutions quite extensively since 1978 without adverse reaction. All TPN patients with documented iron deficiency anemia who are stable and do not require transfusions to repair gross blood loss are candidates for intravenous iron-dextran supplementation. Patients accepted for therapy must have a documented low serum iron, cell indices compatible with microcytic hypo-chromic anemia, and must have demonstrated im-provement in their nutritional status prior to the initiation of therapy. The iron requirement needed to correct the serum hemoglobin is determined from available charts or calculated from the formula [0.3 x body weight in pounds x (100 minus the patient's hemoglobin in grams%) x 100] divided by 14.8 = mg of total iron to be injected. To calculate the dose in ml of iron-dextran (Imferon), the total milligrams must be divided by 50 as 1 ml of Imferon contains 50 mg of iron.

Once the dose has been calculated, 0.5 ml of iron-dex-tran (25 mg of iron) is added to one liter of TPN solution. This bag is hung during a period when Nutrition Support Team is available should adverse reactions occur. Iron-dextran solution will discolor the TPN solution to a rust color. Bags of solution should be checked for precipita-tion prior to hanging. Providing the test dose of iron-dex-tran is well tolerated, 2 ml of iron-dextran (100 mg iron) is added to each succeeding liter of TPN until the calculated dose is administered. The hemoglobin, hematocrit, reti-culocyte count, and transferrin are determined prior to treatment, at weekly intervals during treatment, and one month following treatment to determine the effective-ness of iron-loading therapy. Our experience in over 50 patients has proven this therapy to be safe and effective in correcting the anemia. Iron-dextran therapy has been used in many patients with collagen disorders and only two patients have had symptoms referrable to the ther-apy: one with fever and one with joint pains suggestive of serum sickness. A liver biopsy performed in a home hyperalimentation patient receiving daily Imferon (50 mg of iron) demonstrated large quantities of iron stored in the liver. Since then, iron-dextran has been administered at much lower doses (0.5 ml of iron-dextran, or 25 mg iron on a weekly basis) until the hemoglobin has been restored to normal levels and is then discontinued.

9/Fluid, Electrolytes, and Acid-Base Balance

Introduction and Definition of Terms

Management of fluid, electrolyte, and acid-balance problems is an essential element in an often complex therapeutic plan. The ability of the clinician to deal effectively with fluid replacement, correction of acid-base disorders, and infusion of appropriate electrolytes may determine the success of further therapeutic efforts.

Multiple fluid and electrolyte replacement formulas are available. Each is based on the author's experience and has been developed to meet the needs of others in similar roles. The fluid replacement method presented here has evolved from clinical experiences obtained on a Nutrition Support Service which has been responsible for the intravenous fluid management of its patients since 1976. This method has been developed for the adult patient and is not intended for pediatric or neonatal use. Although an effort has been made to provide practical formulas for fluid replacement and correction of acid-base disorders, they are not intended to replace sound clinical judgement.

A general overview and definition of terms are necessary for a clear understanding of the management of fluids, electrolytes, and acid-base disorders. The following definitions are provided as a baseline.

Total Body Water

Total body water (TBW) makes up 60% of body weight in young men and 55% in young women. TBW content varies considerably, depending upon muscle mass which is associated with increased amounts of body water and fat content which contains much less water per unit volume.

Females have lesser amounts of TBW than males, and infants and children have increased amounts of TBW due to differences in body composition, i.e. muscle mass vs. fat stores. A 15% variation in TBW is possible based on these factors. In some very thin or very obese patients, the TBW may exceed these variations.

Body Weight

Body weight is a key element in the management of any patient on IV fluids. It is used to identify fluid shifts and adequate fluid replacement. Body weights should be determined using the same scale each day to insure accuracy. Conversion of body weight to kilograms is necessary when calculating fluid replacement. Kilograms can be determined by the following formula:

$$\frac{\text{Weight in pounds}}{2.2} = \text{Kg}$$

Extracellular Fluid

The extracellular fluid is composed of two major fluid compartments: *interstitial fluid* which makes up 15% of body weight, and *plasma* which is equivalent to 5% of body weight. The total extracellular fluid compartment amounts to 20% of body weight. Transfer of fluids between these compartments is rapid and may be in excess of 500 ml per hour with loss of plasma volume or loading with IV fluids. Similar shifts from the interstitial to plasma space can be identified with volume loss due to the aggressive use of diuretics.

The electrolyte composition of interstitial fluid should be considered equivalent to serum levels, i.e. Na 144, K 4, Ca 3, Mg 2, Cl 103, bicarbonate 27, phosphate 3, organic acids, and protein 6 (mEq/L).

Blood Volume

Blood volume can be calculated as 7-8% of body weight. The plasma represents 5% of body weight, and red blood cells contribute another 2-3%.

Intracellular Fluid

The intracellular water represents 30-40% of body weight, with the majority of this fluid located within the skeletal muscle cells. With dehydration, intracellular fluid diffuses into the interstitial fluid compartment where it may be shifted to the intravascular space to maintain circulatory volume. Similarly, overhydration causes a shift of fluid from the interstitial space into the cells, expanding their total water content.

Osmolarity

Normal serum osmolarity is 285 ± 15 milliosmoles. The osmolarity represents the number of particles (millimoles) dissolved in one liter of water. The electrolytes contribute greatly to the osmolarity of plasma. Each molecule is responsible for one millimole i.e. sodium, potassium, and chloride. Multivalent elements, i.e. calcium, phosphate, and magnesium, provide one millimole for each molecule represented. Thus, calcium chloride ($CaCl_2$) provides 3 millimoles.

Urea, glucose, and proteins provide one milliosmole for each molecule contained in the solution. Plasma proteins are responsible for the colloid osmotic pressure but, because of their large molecular size, are not readily diffused into the interstitial fluid. Thus, an osmotic gradient is provided in the capillaries which returns the diffusable fluid and electrolytes to the venous system for return to the heart.

Serum osmolarity can be calculated from the following equation:

$$\text{Osmolarity} = 2 \times (Na^+ + K^+) + \frac{BUN}{2.8} + \frac{Glucose}{18}$$

Fluid Replacement

In normal circumstances, oral intake of fluids provides the most efficient and effective method of replacing volume losses. In surgical patients, the oral route is frequently interrupted or defunctionalized to the point that intravenous fluids must be used to maintain equilibrium within the body. During these periods when oral intake is interrupted, a rational plan for fluid replacement must be initiated.

Fluid Losses

Fluid losses are classically described as insensible or sensible. Insensible fluid losses are usually not measured. These losses occur as a result of evaporation of water from the skin and water vapor loss through respiration. In carefully balanced studies, the insensible loss spans a wide range from 500-1000 ml per day, depending upon body size, body temperature, and ambient conditions.

Insensible Fluid Loss

Lungs	25%	200-300 ml
Skin	75%	400-600 ml

Sensible losses represent measurable losses of fluid volume through urine, stool, tubes, and fistulas. Although minimal urinary output of 20-30 ml/hour may be acceptable in some circumstances, greater volumes of urine are desired to provide leeway for individuals with marginal renal function in which the ability to concentrate urine may be less than optimal. Thus, urine output of 480-720 ml/24 hours could be acceptable, but a more desirable urinary output would be in the range of 1200-1500 ml, thereby reducing the need for maximum urine concentration and optimal renal tubular function.

Losses of fluids into the stool in the non-diarrhea setting amount to 100-150 ml per day. This loss is usually considered equivalent to the water gained from the metabolic process when glucose is metabolized to carbon dioxide and water. When diarrhea is present, every effort must be made to measure stool losses to insure adequate fluid replacement.

Third Space Fluid Losses

Third space fluid loss is a term applied to volume losses within the body which cannot be measured under most conditions. Examples of third space fluid include intraperitoneal fluid associated with peritonitis. Fluid losses due to generalized peritonitis have been estimated to be equivalent to a 30% body burn. Replacement can be calculated according to the Baxter Burn Formula:

4 ml x % burn (30%) x weight in Kg = volume lost.

Other examples of third space losses include bowel obstruction where massive amounts of fluid are contained within the bowel, ileofemoral thrombosis where tissue fluids are sequestered into the lower extremities, pancreatitis where large amounts of fluid are transudated into the retroperitoneal space, and burns where edema fluid in large quantities permeates the burn area.

Attempts to estimate third space fluid losses are difficult, and weight changes may often be the only measurable data. With the development of third space retention, volume replacement must be initiated to maintain effective circulating volume.

Calculating Volume Replacement

Replacing volume on the basis of insensible and measured volume losses is open to great variability due to body size, age of the patient, and the presence or absence of third space fluid retention. In an effort to correlate fluid replacement needs with body size, the following guideline can be used in patients with minimal third space fluid retention:

34-45 ml/Kg/24 hours

This guideline provides some assistance in planning fluid replacement for a 90 year old, 80-pound patient vs. a 220-pound 20 year old football player. Clearly, the usual 2500-3000 ml of IV fluids might be hazardous to the small elderly patient, yet provide insufficient replacement to the robust athlete.

Monitoring Fluid Replacement

Monitoring fluid replacement will depend on the clinical problem, associated disease processes, and fragility of the patient. Fluid replacement in the young or middle-aged patient following elective operative procedures may require little concern, whereas large volume replacements for the elderly with associated heart problems, renal disease, or closed head injury may require the ultimate in monitoring.

The first stage of fluid monitoring includes close observation of vital signs, i.e. blood pressure, pulse, respiration, and temperature. Periodic evaluation of the lungs for overhydration will add to your clinical assessment of fluid replacement.

The second stage of fluid monitoring includes observation of urinary output. Frequently, a urinary catheter becomes a necessity, and hourly readings or fractions thereof may prove essential to the regulation of volume replacement. Urine specific gravity may be used to determine hemo-concentration states, and a comparison of urine osmolarity to serum osmolarity may prove helpful.

The third stage of fluid monitoring includes central venous pressure readings to insure adequate volume return to the heart. A central line inserted via the subclavian route or internal jugular with documentation of the catheter tip at the level of the right atrium may be necessary in those patients in whom urinary output is adequate and volume replacement is in doubt. Central venous pressures below 5 usually suggest inadequate replacement, and central venous pressure above 15 suggests adequate volume replacement and should be of concern if an increase in IV infusions is under consideration.

The fourth stage of fluid monitoring involves the placement of a Swan-Ganz catheter into the pulmonary vascular tree to measure end-diastolic, left atrial pressure. In complicated resuscitation problems, the Swan-Ganz catheter is extremely effective as a measure of the cardiac response and can provide additional information regarding cardiac output, peripheral resistance, and other hemodynamic measurements which may impact heavily upon volume replacement and other resuscitative measures.

Volume Deficits

In controlled environments, i.e. hospitals or where strict intake and output has been recorded, volume deficiencies can be calculated and replaced precisely. Where gastrointestinal losses have occurred, estimates of the electrolyte composition for specific losses have been determined.

GASTROINTESTINAL LOSSES

Source	Sodium	Potassium	Chloride
Gastric	59.0	9.3	89.0
Upper Small Bowel	104.9	5.1	98.9
Ileum	116.7	5.0	105.8
Bile	145.3	5.2	99.9
Pancreatic Juice	141.6	4.6	76.6

Although fluid and electrolyte replacement can be accomplished on the basis of this information, a more desirable method is to determine the electrolyte composition in fluid losses that exceed 300-500 ml/day. Aliquots of these solutions can be sent to the lab for an electrolyte determination. With these results, specific solutions can be tailored to meet the losses of both fluid and electrolytes. The necessity for determining electrolytes in fluid losses rests heavily on the fact that most fluid losses are a combination of gastrointestinal losses, with great individual variability in electrolyte composition.

Where volume losses have occurred and adequate measurement is lacking, i.e. vomiting or diarrhea at home or the accumulation of large amounts of third space fluid, clinical assessment of volume losses becomes an essential part in planning the replacement program. A classification of dehydration based on symptoms and clinical findings may be extremely useful in these circumstances.

Mild Dehydration: 4-6% loss of body weight

Mild dehydration is frequently manifested by a feeling

of thirst and a history of decreased or concentrated urinary output. Clinical findings include dry mucous membranes, stable vital signs, and a loss of skin turgor.

Moderate Dehydration: 8% loss of body weight

Moderate dehydration is manifested by a feeling of thirst, apathy, orthostatic hypotension, tachycardia, collapsed veins, decreased skin turgor, and a weak pulse.

Severe Dehydration: 10% loss of body weight

Severe dehydration is identified by stupor or coma, hypotension in a reclining position, soft sunken eyes, absent or decreased urinary output, cold extremities, and absent or weak peripheral pulses.

Replacement of Dehydration Losses

When volume replacement is indicated, there are a number of IV fluids available, each with a different pH and electrolyte composition.

VOLUME REPLACEMENT FLUIDS

Solution	pH	Na	K	Cl	Ca	Glucose	Lactate
Normal Saline (0.9 NaCl)	5.0	155	–	155	–	–	–
D$_5$ NS	4.5	155	–	155	–	270	–
D$_5$ ½NS (D$_5$ 0.45 NaCl)	4.0	78	–	78	–	270	–
D$_5$ ¼NS	4.0	39	–	39	–	270	–

Ringer's Lactate	6.5	130	4	109	3	–	28
D_5 RL	5.0	130	4	109	3	270	28

Dehydration losses represent a loss of extracellular fluid and should be replaced with Ringer's lactate solution, usually without dextrose. The dehydration losses must be replaced in addition to the usual maintenance requirement of fluid. Thus, a 154-pound (70 Kg) patient with severe dehydration (10% loss) should receive 7 liters of Ringer's lactate solution. Should the patient require operative intervention, 50% of the calculated fluid loss should be replaced prior to surgery.

When an operative procedure is not indicated, fluid replacement can be conducted over a 48-hour period by replacing 2/3 of the calculated fluid loss within the first 24 hours and the final 1/3 during the second 24 hours. Under these circumstances, the patient should have received an additional 2.5 liters of fluid per day to replace the usual fluid requirements. Thus, the total volume replacement during the first 24 hours should be 4.7 or 5 liters of Ringer's lactate plus 2.5 liters of half-normal saline. IV replacement on the second day would amount to 2.5 liters of Ringer's lactate plus 2.5 liters of half-normal saline.

Monitoring fluid replacement in this patient would require careful observation of vital signs, pulmonary auscultation, urinary catheterization, and usually, central venous pressure monitoring.

Overhydration

Although overhydration can be a problem, the presence of edema does not assure adequate intravascular volume. Patients may require additional intravenous volume replacement in spite of obvious peripheral edema. With stabilization, diuresis will ensue, and the third space fluid manifested as edema will resolve. Little would be gained by using diuretics in the early resuscitative period. In fact, forced diuresis may precipitate renal failure which carries an overall mortality rate of 60% in the post-operative patient.

Electrolyte Replacement

Electrolyte loss through the skin is minimal under normal circumstances where 400-600 ml of fluid is lost via evaporation. Ten to 60 mEq of NaCl is associated with this loss. With profuse sweating, 100-150 mEq NaCl/L may be lost via the skin.

The functioning kidney has remarkable capacities to retain sodium and fluid under most circumstances. The kidneys may reabsorb all but 5-10 mEq of sodium per day when under the influence of aldosterone. Normal oral intake of sodium varies from 75-120 mEq per day. In the uncomplicated post-operative patient, 75-150 mEq of sodium should be replaced on a daily basis. This is equivalent to 1725-3450 mg of sodium, or 4.5-9.0 gm of salt. *Conversion of mEq to mg of sodium* is performed as follows:

$$\text{mEq Na} \times 23 = \text{mg Na}$$

The following formula will *convert mg of sodium into grams of salt* (NaCl):

$$\frac{\text{mg Na}}{.38} = \frac{\text{mg salt}}{1000} = \text{grams salt}$$

The kidney's ability to conserve potassium is less efficient. An obligatory loss of 30-40 mEq/day can be expected, even when oral or IV intake is zero. Thus, potassium replacement of 60-90 mEq per day should be implemented. In the early post-operative period, potassium is released from the cells with the development of increased potassium levels in the extracellular fluid. Therefore, potassium should be withheld from intravenous fluids for the first 24 hours following stress (trauma or operation) unless a serum potassium level is obtained or adequate urinary output is assured.

Based on this information, *a simple guideline to electrolyte replacement is as follows:*

1. Replace 2 mEq of sodium per Kg per day.
2. Replace 1 mEq of potassium per Kg per day *after* the first post-operative day where urinary output has been documented.

The addition of magnesium, calcium, and other electrolytes is not necessary in the usual post-operative patient, but may become a vital concern if the patient is receiving nutritional support where replenishment of the intracellular electrolytes is essential (calcium, magnesium, phosphate, and potassium).

Special Fluid and Electrolyte Problems

Hyperkalemia

Hyperkalemia is associated with the multiple causes of metabolic acidosis, including diabetic ketoacidosis, renal failure, and occasionally, post-resuscitative metabolic acidosis. Serum potassium levels of 7 mEq/L developing on an acute basis can be responsible for cardiac arrest. Potassium levels of 6 mEq/L should be considered dangerous and therapy immediately initiated to reduce it to normal levels.

Correction of the underlying metabolic cause of acidosis is frequently adequate to reduce elevated serum potassium levels. Other measures include infusion of glucose and insulin solutions which will drive the potassium intracellularly, and chelating compounds such as Kayexalate which can be used orally or as enemas to reduce hyperpotassemia. Dialysis can be used effectively, but carries the risk of establishing vascular access.

Hypokalemia

When replacing potassium, caution should be used with intravenous infusions containing more than 30-40 mEq per liter. A standard rule of thumb is that no more than 40 mEq potassium may be infused per hour. At this level, cardiac arrest may occur; thus, when infusing large volumes of potassium, cardiac monitoring as well as repeated serum electrolyte levels are necessary to insure patient safety.

Fluid Retention with Ascites and Edema

The syndrome of fluid retention with an associated low serum sodium almost always represents an underlying chronic process such as hepatic cirrhosis, ovarian carcinoma or other neoplasms with peritoneal implantations, or congestive heart failure resulting from constricting pericarditis or cardiac insufficiency. Although the patient has excessive total body water, the intravascular volume is often deficient due to the peritoneal leak. The hypo-volemia stimulates the release of renin, angiotensin, and aldosterone hormones, which increases sodium and water retention. The serum sodium in many of these patients will reach as low as 115-120 mEq/liter and, be-cause of the chronicity of the problem, will have little, if any, associated CNS effects. The body has, in effect, re-established a much lower sodium status in which it is able to function. Establishing a therapeutic program for these patients involves three objectives:

1. Withholding all sodium and markedly restricting fluids.
2. Elimination of excess fluids, i.e. IV medications.
3. Correction of the underlying disease process.

The combination of sodium and fluid restriction along with the judicious use of diuretics can be effective when coupled with the appropriate use of chemotherapy agents or nutritional support.

Inappropriate ADH Syndrome

The syndrome of inappropriate ADH is associated with chronically ill patients having low serum sodium and fluid retention. Most of these patients will not have significant ascites and, although edema may be present, it is usually of lesser significance. The distinguishing features of this syndrome are the dilutional hyponatremia with low serum osmolarity and a highly concentrated urine osmo-larity with high sodium concentrations. Serum sodium below 126 is frequently associated with muscular twitch-ing, hyperactive tendon reflexes, convulsions, and signs of increased intracranial pressure. When CNS signs prevail, hypertonic sodium chloride (3%) can be used judiciously. However, in most circumstances, marked fluid restriction will correct the problem in short order.

Acid-Base Disorders

Electrolyte abnormalities are frequently the first indication of acid-base disorders. Ventilatory problems should signal the procurement of arterial blood gases which will also reveal acid-base abnormalities. The combination of these two labortory tests should readily identify the acid-base problem when one considers the underlying medical/surgical problem.

The normal pH of arterial blood is 7.38 to 7.42. To understand acid-base disorders, it is important to realize that there are three basic mechanisms to maintain a stable pH. Blood is capable of buffering the pH through its protein concentration and serum bicarbonate. The major buffering capacity of blood resides in the hemoglobin of the red cells. In most circumstances, this buffering mechanism is sufficient to maintain a stable equilibrium in spite of large quantities of acid generation through metabolism.

The second mechanism for buffering pH resides in the pulmonary capacity to remove excess hydrogen ion as water and CO_2 through the acetic acid equilibrium:

$$HCO_3^- + H^+ \rightleftharpoons H_2O + CO_2$$

H_2CO_3 is unique in that it has a high endogenous production, and the concentration is regulated by respiration. Thus, disturbances of a respiratory nature will be noted by an increasing or decreasing pCO_2 concentration. The renal excretion of electrolytes, acid, and base provides the final buffering mechanism for a stable arterial pH.

Normally, these three buffering mechanisms work together to maintain a stable pH in the body.

Interpretation of arterial blood gases can be confusing; however, when dealing with acid-base disorders, only three factors are important. The pH indicates the acid or base status of arterial blood. Readings higher than 7.42 indicate alkalosis, results below 7.38 indicate acidosis. The blood has an efficient buffering capacity, and the respiratory and renal systems can make appropriate adjustments to counteract the internal acid or alkaline environment. Therefore, the pH often does not reflect the true hydrogen ion concentration and be interpreted as:

> *Uncompensated acidosis or alkalosis:* little or no evidence of respiratory or renal adjustment to correct the abnormal acid or alkalotic state.

> *Partially compensated acidosis or alkalosis:* respiratory and renal adjustments have been initiated, but of insufficient magnitude to correct the pH to normal limits.

> *Fully compensated acidosis or alkalosis:* respiratory and renal adjustments have been able to correct the pH to normal values.

The following equation can be used to assist in determining the degree of compensation:

$$H^+ \text{ concentration} = \frac{24 \times pCO_2}{HCO_3^-}$$

The hydrogen ion concentration for uncompensated pH values are listed below.

CONVERSION OF pH to H$^+$ CONCENTRATION

pH		H$^+$	pH		H$^+$	pH		H$^+$	pH		H$^+$
7.10	=	79	7.32	=	49	7.38	=	42	7.44	=	37
7.15	=	71	7.34	=	48	7.39	=	41	7.46	=	36
7.20	=	63	7.35	=	46	7.40	=	40	7.48	=	34
7.25	=	57	7.36	=	44	7.41	=	39	7.50	=	32
7.30	=	50	7.37	=	43	7.42	=	38	7.60	=	25

A normal pH of 7.4 has a H$^+$ concentration of 40. Thus, the pCO_2 can be determined if the HCO_3^- is known:

$$40 = \frac{24 \times CO_2}{27} = pCO_2 \text{ of } 15$$

The pCO_2 listed on the arterial blood gas report indicates the respiratory component of the acid base problem and may reflect the primary problem or a compensatory mechanism for a metabolic problem. *Base excess or deficit* reported on arterial blood gases likewise reflects the metabolic component. Deficits indicate retained fixed acids, i.e. organic acids such as lactic acid, ketoacidosis, or accumulation of acid products of metabolism ($pO_4^=$ or $SO_4^=$). Base excess indicates a loss of hydrogen ion or an accumulation of base such as bicarbonate or citrate through exogenous infusion or renal reabsorption. Although the pO_2 listed on the arterial blood gas report does not determine acid-base status, it may help identify the primary problem and is vital to cellular metabolism.

Anion gap is frequently useful in determining the quantity of fixed acid responsible in metabolic acidosis and can be calculated as follows:

Anion Gap = $Na^+ - Cl^-$

Example: Na=143 mEq and Cl=103 mEq; 143 – 103 = 40 mEq/L

The *predicted standard bicarbonate* can be computed from the anion gap:

Anion Gap ÷ 1.6 = predicted standard bicarbonate

Example: 40 ÷ 1.6 = 25 mEq/L = predicted standard bicarbonate

The *unaccounted anion* is determined from the predicted standard bicarbonate minus the actual bicarbonate level.

Example: An elderly gentleman is admitted with a small bowel obstruction. Electrolytes are Na 145 mEq, Cl 90 mEq, HCO_3 15 mEq/L.

145 – 90 = 55 (Anion Gap)

55 ÷ 1.6 = 34.3 (Predicted standard bicarbonate)

34.3 – 15 (actual bicarbonate) = 19.3 (Unaccounted anion)

Assessment: 19.3 mEq anion is probably lactic acid due to anaerobic metabolism and hypovolemia.

Respiratory Acidosis

Respiratory acidosis resulting from inadequate ventilation should precipitate a search for the factors responsible, i.e. narcotic overdose, inadequate ventilation following anesthesia (too early extubation), pneumothorax or pleural effusion, atelectasis (aspiration, accumulation of secretions), or pulmonary embolism. Appropriate use of ventilators, drugs, or pain control (intercostal nerve blocks) should be initiated to correct the problem.

Respiratory Alkalosis

Respiratory alkalosis may represent CNS stimulation associated with shock or trauma, or it may represent inadequate dead space or over-ventilation of the patient on a respirator. Appropriate addition of greater dead space or re-setting the ventilator will usually correct this problem.

Metabolic Acidosis

Metabolic acidosis occurs frequently with shock, dehydration, and sepsis. Adequate volume replacement is the key to correcting this problem. If volume replacement should fail to correct metabolic acidosis, sodium bicarbonate is generally effective. The *bicarbonate space* within the body has been calculated at 30% of the total body weight. Thus, the bicarbonate deficit can be determined from the serum electrolyte x 30% x weight in Kg.

For example, a patient with a small bowel obstruction has the following electrolytes after initial resuscitative measures: Na 142, Cl 103, K 3.9, and HCO_3 15. The patient weighs 75 Kg. Correction would be calculated as follows:

Normal serum bicarbonate of 25 less 15 = 10 mM deficit. 10 x .30 x 75 = 225 mM sodium bicarbonate deficit.

Bicarbonate is available in ampules of 50 mEq, thus the patient should receive 4½ ampules to correct the metabolic acidosis.

Metabolic Alkalosis

Metabolic alkalosis is being noted with increasing frequency in surgical patients. The compensatory mechanisms within the body are least effective in correcting metabolic alkalosis. In addition, the alkalotic state shifts the oxyhemoglobin curve to the left, which impairs oxygen delivery to the tissues. Thus, correction is an essential part of surgical therapy.

Causes of metabolic alkalosis are the loss of hydrogen ion, usually as a result of high output from nasogastric suction or diuretics, or the infusion of large amounts of base. Correction is usually accomplished with infusion of sodium chloride or potassium chloride. On occasions where these solutions do not provide correction, hydrochloric acid can be infused via a central line, preferably with amino acids, i.e. TPN which will buffer the acid effectively. Calculation of HCl replacement is similar to the bicarbonate replacement formula. The bicarbonate excess is determined from the serum electrolytes or arterial blood gases (base excess), and appropriate amounts of HCl are infused according to the same formula.

For example, a 75 Kg patient has persistent metabolic alkalosis as represented by Na 144, Cl 85, K 4.0, HCO_3 35. The bicarbonate excess can be calculated by determining the difference between a normal serum bicarbonate of 25 and the recorded value of 35, in this case an excess of 10 mEq. 10 x .30 x 75 = 225 mEq of HCl would be required to correct this problem.

Summary

This brief overview of the management of fluid, electrolyte, and acid-base disorders is designed to provide a practical working knowledge of the usual problems encountered. An inquisitive mind and diligent effort to seek out answers from the medical literature will be necessary to resolve the more complex problems that can arise in the clinical setting.

10/Summary

A standard protocol for total parenteral nutrition can serve as a basis for establishing a safe and efficient TPN system in most any institution, irrespective of size or degree of nutritional expertise. A pragmatic approach to identification and selection of the TPN patient and the proper placement of a central venous catheter via the subclavian route is essential. The efficacy of standard solutions and their adaptation to various clinical problems should provide a workable guideline for most institutions. Careful attention to patient monitoring and appropriate additions or alterations of the TPN solution permits adaptability to meet individual patient needs and allows for early adjustments which will deter many of the complex metabolic problems which in the past have led to early discontinuation of therapy. The use of TPN to support the metabolic and nutritionally depleted patient carries considerable risk which can be substantially reduced by a well-organized TPN program.

Tables

TABLE I: Comparison of Indirect Calorimetry to Various REE Estimates

Patient	HBE	HBE + Long's	25 kcal/kg	35 kcal/kg	Wilmore
Surgery	NS	p<0.01	p<0.01	p<0.01	p<0.01
Cancer	NS	p<0.01	NS	p<0.01	
Surgery & Cancer	NS	p<0.01	NS	p<0.01	
Surgery & Sepsis	NS	p<0.01	NS	p<0.01	
Skeletal Trauma	NS	p<0.01	NS	p<0.01	p<0.01
No Stress Factor	NS		NS	p<0.01	
Ventilator Patients	NS	p<0.01	NS	p<0.01	

TABLE II: Comparison of Subclavian Catheter Studies

	1977-78 (6 mos)	1979-80 (18 mos)
Number of Patients	46	337
Number of Catheters	49	397
Malpositioned	3 (6.1%)	18 (4.5%)
Failure to Place	6 (12.2%)	23 (5.8%)
Sepsis	1 (2.0%)	4 (1.0%)
Pneumothorax	3 (6.1%)	9 (2.3%)
Changed over Guidewire	0	28 (7.1%)

TABLE III: Patient Monitoring

1. Daily weights.

2. Blood sugars, BUN, and electrolytes daily X3 or until stable, then every Monday-Wednesday-Friday.

3. CBC with differential, transferrin, Mg^{++}, and SMA drawn on Day 1 and weekly thereafter; Serum zinc level drawn prior to initiation of TPN solutions.

4. Urine for sugar and acetone every 6 hours using Ketodiastix.

TABLE IV: TPN Solution A

1 L contains 42.5 gms protein, 6.8 gms N and 850 non-N cals.
Cal:Gms N=125:1.

Travasol 8.5% with lytes	500ml	Electrolyte Composition:	
Dextrose 50%	500ml	Na	35 mEq
Calcium Gluconate	4.5mEq	K	30 mEq
		Acetate	65 mEq
May add (specify):		Mg	5 mEq
1. Electrolytes		Cl	35 mEq
2. Standard Additives		PO$_4$	30 mEq
(MVI and Trace minerals 1 cc)		Ca	4.5 mEq

3. May change Dextrose concentration by writing TPN Sol A(D___)

TABLE V: TPN Solution B

1 L contains 42.5 gms protein, 6.8 gms N and 850 non-N cals.
Cal:Gms N=125:1.

Travasol 8.5% s̄ lytes	500ml	Electrolyte Composition:	
Dextrose 50%	500ml	Acetate	26 mEq
		Cl	17 mEq

May add (specify):
1. Electrolytes
2. Standard Additives
3. May change Dextrose concentration by writing TPN Sol B(D___)

TABLE VI: Solution E

1 L contains 27.5 gms protein, 4.4 gms N and 850 non-N cals.
Cal:Gms N=193:1.

		Electrolyte Composition:	
Travasol 5.5% with lytes	500ml		
Dextrose 50%	500ml	Na	35 mEq
Calcium Gluconate	4.5mEq	K	30 mEq
		Mg	5 mEq
May add (specify):		Acetate	50 mEq
1. Electrolytes		Cl	35 mEq
2. Standard Additives		PO$_4$	30 mEq
		Ca	4.5 mEq

3. May change Dextrose concentration by writing TPN Sol E(D___)

TABLE VII: Solution F

1 L contains 27.5 gms protein, 4.4 gms N and 850 non-N cals.
Cal:Gms N=193:1.

		Electrolyte Composition:	
Travasol 5.5% s̄ lytes	500ml		
Dextrose 50%	500ml	Acetate	17 mEq
		Cl	11 mEq

May add, decrease, or delete (specify):
1. Electrolytes
2. May change Dextrose concentration by writing TPN Sol F(D___)

TABLE VIII: Solution D (Surgery Solution)

1 L contains 42.5 gms protein, 6.8 gms N and 340 non-N cals.
Cal:Gms N=50:1.

Travasol 8.5% s̄ lytes	500ml	Electrolyte Composition:	
Dextrose 20%	500ml	Acetate	26 mEq
		Cl	17 mEq

May add (specify):
1. Electrolytes
2. Standard Additives
NOTE: To be used 6 hours pre-op and for 24-48 hours post-op.

TABLE IX: Solution S-1

625 cc contains 10.62 gms protein, 1.7 gms N and 850 non-N cals.
Cal:Gms N=500:1.

Travasol 8.5% s̄ lytes	125ml	Electrolyte Composition:	
Dextrose 50%	500ml	Acetate	6.5 mEq
		Cl	4 mEq

May add (specify):
1. Electrolytes
2. Standard Additives
3. May change Dextrose concentration by writing TPN Sol S-1(D___)

TABLE X: Solution S-2

750 cc contains 21.25 gms protein, 3.4 gms N and 850 non-N cals.
Cal:Gms N=250:1.

Travasol 8.5% s̄ lytes	250ml	Electrolyte Composition:	
Dextrose 50%	500ml	Acetate	13 mEq
		Cl	8 mEq

May add (specify):
1. Electrolytes
2. Standard Additives
3. May change Dextrose concentration by writing TPN Sol S-2(D___)

TABLE XI: Solution for Pulmonary Failure

850 ml contains 42.5 gms protein, 6.8 gms N and 833 non-N cals.
Cal:Gms N=222:1.

Travasol 8.5% s̄ lytes	500ml	Electrolyte Composition:	
Dextrose 70%	350ml	Na	35 mEq
		K	30 mEq
May add (as required):		Acetate	65 mEq
1. Electrolytes		Mg	5 mEq
2. Standard Additives		Cl	35 mEq
		PO₄	30 mEq
Lipid 20% (infused separately): 360 ml		Ca	4.5 mEq

TABLE XII: Solution for Fluid Overload Syndromes

1 L contains 42.5 gms protein, 6.8 gms N and 1200 non-N cals.
Cal:Gms N=176:1.

Travasol 8.5% s lytes	500ml	Electrolyte Composition:	
Dextrose 70%	500ml	Acetate	26 mEq
		Cl	17 mEq

Add:
30 mEq KCl
8 meq MgSO$_4$
4.5 mEq Calcium gluconate
Standard Additives (MVI 12 and trace minerals)
Electrolytes

TABLE XIII: MVI-12 Multi-Vitamin Infusion Solution®

MVI-12 Vial 1 (5 ml) provides:

Ascorbic acid (C) .... 100 mg
Vitamin A (retinol) .... 3,300 IU
Vitamin D (ergocalciferol) .... 200 IU
Thiamine HCl (B1) .... 3.0 mg
Riboflavin-5-phosphate (B2)........................ 3.6 mg
Pyridoxine HCl (B6) .... 4.0 mg
Niacinamide .... 40.0 mg
Pantothenic acid .... 15.0 mg
Vitamin E .... 10 IU

MVI-12 Vial 2 (5 ml) provides:

Biotin .... 60 mcg
Folic acid .... 400 mcg
Vitamin B12 .... 5 mcg

TABLE XIV: IMS Multiple Trace Metal Additive®

1 ml contains:	Manganese	0.5 mg
	Copper	1.0 mg
	Zinc	4.0 mg
	Chromium	10 mcg

References

1. Cowan, G. and Sheetz, W.: *Intravenous Hyperalimentation.* Philadelphia, 1972, Lea & Febiger, pp. v-x.

2. Meng, H.C.: Parenteral Nutrition: Principles, nutrient requirements, techniques, and clinical applications. In Schneider, H.A., Anderson, C.E., and Coursin, D.B. (eds.): *Nutritional Support of Medical Practice.* Hagerstown, 1977, Harper and Row, pp. 152-176.

3. Fischer, J.E.: *Total Parenteral Nutrition.* Boston, 1976, Little, Brown and Company, p. xi.

4. Blackburn, G.L., Bistrian B.R., Maini B.S., et al: Nutritional and metabolic assessment of the hospitalized patient. J. Parenteral Enteral Nutr. 1:11-12, 1977.

5. Mullen, J.L.: Prediction of operative morbidity and mortality by preoperative nutritional assessment. Surg. Forum 39:80-82, 1979.

6. Miller, S.F., Finley, R.K. and Morath, M.A.: Derivation of serum transferrin. JAMA 246:39, 1981.

7. Petersen, D.P., Gilbert, M.L. and Dean, R.E.: Transferrin as a predictor of mortality in the parenterally alimented patient. Unpublished manuscript.

8. Grant, A.: *Nutritional Assessment Guidelines.* Berkeley, 1979, Cutter Medical Company.

9. Harris, J.A. and Benedict, F.G.: *Biometric Studies of Basal Metabolism in Man.* Washington DC, 1919, Carnegie Institute of Washington, Pub 279.

10. Fischer, J.E., Funovics, J.M., Aguirre, A., et al: The role of plasma amino acids in hepatic encephalopathy. Surgery 78:276-290, 1975.

11. Abel, R.M., Beck, C.H., Abbott, W.W., et al: Treatment of acute renal failure with intravenous administration of essential amino acids and glucose. Surg. Forum 23:77-79, 1972.

12. Dudrick, S.J., Steiger, E. and Long, J.M.: Renal failure in surgical patients: Treatment with intravenous essential amino acids and hypertonic glucose. Surgery 68:180-186, 1970.

13. Fishberg, A.M.: *Hypertension and Nephritis,* ed 5. Philadelphia, 1954, Lea & Febiger, p. 266.

14. Giovannetti, S. and Maggiore, Q.: A low nitrogen diet with proteins of high biological value for severe chronic uremia. Lancet 1:1000-1003, 1964.

15. Fell, G.S. and Burns, R.R.: Zinc and other trace elements. In Ivan, D.A. Johnston (ed): *Advances in Parenteral Nutrition.* Lancaster, England, 1978, MTP Press Ltd., pp. 245-259.

16. Kartinos, N.J.: Trace element formulations in intravenous feeding. In Ivan, D.A. Johnston (ed.): *Advances in Parenteral Nutrition.* Lancaster, England, 1978, MTP Press Ltd., pp. 233-240.

17. Broviac, J.W., Cole, B.S. and Scribner, B.H.: A silicone rubber atrial catheter for prolonged parenteral alimentation. Surg. Gynecol. and Obstet. 136:1-5, 1973.

18. Dudrick, S.J., Wilmore, D.W., Vars, H.M., et al: Can intravenous feeding as the sole means of nutrition support growth in the child and restore weight loss in an adult? An affirmative answer. In *Transactions of the Southern Surgical Association,* Vol LXXX. Philadelphia, J.B. Lippincott Company, 1969, pp. 370-380.

19. Kaminski, M.V. and Sriram, K.: *A New Catheter for Home Enteral Hyperalimentation* (monograph), Chicago, 1981, pp. 1-6.

20. Heimbach, D.M. and Ivey, T.D.: Technique for placement of a permanent home hyperalimentation catheter. Surg. Gynecol. and Obstet. 143:634-636, 1976.

21. Steiger, E.: TPN Catheterization. In *Clinical Parenteral Nutrition,* Irvine, McGaw Laboratories Publication, 1977, pp. 29-31.

22. Wilson, R.F.: *Fluids, Electrolytes and Metabolism.* Springfield, 1973, Charles C. Thomas, pp. 13-15.

23. Giordano, C., Pluvio, M., and Esposito, R.: Urea index and nitrogen balance in uremic patients on minimal nitrogen intakes. Clin. Nephrol. 3:168-171, 1975.

24. Driver, A.G. and Leg, N.M.: Iatrogenic malnutrition in patients receiving ventilatory support. JAMA 244:2195-2196, 1980.

25. Askanazi, J., Elwyn, D.H., Silverburg, P.A. et al: Respiratory distress secondary to a high carbohydrate load: A case report. Surgery 87:596-598, 1980.

26. Vanderween, T.W.: Drug-nutrition interrelationships—An expanded role for the nutritional support team pharmacist. J. Parenteral Enteral Nutr. 3:5, 1981.

27. Sherman, R.L.: Clinical concepts in potassium therapy. In *Hospital Management* #2, Columbus, ADRIA Laboratories Inc., 1980.

28. Finkle, D. and Dean, R.E.: Buffered hydrochloric acid: A modern method of treating metabolic alkalosis. Am. Surgeon 47:103-106, 1981.

Index

Notes

Notes